THE
TRUE
YOU
DIET

THE
TRUE
YOU
DIET

The revolutionary diet programme that
identifies your unique body chemistry and
reveals the foods that are right for YOU

DR JOHN BRIFFA

HAY HOUSE

Australia • Canada • Hong Kong
South Africa • United Kingdom • United States

First published and distributed in the United Kingdom by:
Hay House UK Ltd, 292B Kensal Rd, London W10 5BE. Tel.: (44) 20 8962 1230;
Fax: (44) 20 8962 1239. www.hayhouse.co.uk

Published and distributed in the United States of America by:
Hay House, Inc., PO Box 5100, Carlsbad, CA 92018–5100. Tel.: (1) 760 431 7695 or (800) 654 5126;
Fax: (1) 760 431 6948 or (800) 650 5115. www.hayhouse.com

Published and distributed in Australia by:
Hay House Australia Ltd, 18/36 Ralph St, Alexandria NSW 2015. Tel.: (61) 2 9669 4299;
Fax: (61) 2 9669 4144. www.hayhouse.com.au

Published and distributed in the Republic of South Africa by:
Hay House SA (Pty), Ltd, PO Box 990, Witkoppen 2068. Tel./Fax: (27) 11 706 6612.
orders@psdprom.co.za

Published and distributed in India by:
Hay House Publishers India, Muskaan Complex, Plot No.3, B-2, Vasant Kunj, New Delhi – 110 070.
Tel.: (91) 11 41761620; Fax: (91) 11 41761630. contact@hayhouseindia.co.in

Distributed in Canada by:
Raincoast, 9050 Shaughnessy St, Vancouver, BC V6P 6E5. Tel.: (1) 604 323 7100;
Fax: (1) 604 323 2600

A catalogue record for this book is available from the British Library.

ISBN 978-1-4019-1543-8

Composition by Scribe Design, Ashford, Kent, UK.
Printed and bound in Great Britain by TJ International, Padstow, Cornwall.

Acknowledgements

Robert Kirby – my agent. For being the most un-agenty agent I've ever met and a lovely bloke to boot.

Michelle Pilley and Jo Burgess of Hay House. Not only for your profession-alism, but for being wonderful people to work with, too.

Joe Briffa – my brother. For reading and commenting constructively on some early drafts of the manuscript, as well as for your enthusiasm, advice and support over the years.

Dr Joseph Briffa – my Dad. For going through my original manuscript with a fine-tooth comb and for showing me the error of my grammatical ways.

Dr Dorothy Burgess – my Mum. For all those things only a mother can offer that I am truly grateful for.

Dr Pete Robbins. Not just for being a brill mate, but also for your sagely advice regarding the scientific aspects of the book.

John 'Fray' Bennett. For concocting some really wonderful 'hunter' recipes, and for ensuring that cooking is always a pleasure and never a chore.

Sera Irvine. Not just for masterminding the delicious 'hunter-gatherer' dishes in this book, but also for your friendship, passion and humour.

Jyotish Patel. For dreaming up the tantalizing 'gatherer' dishes in this book, as well as for being a very special friend.

Andy Metcalfe and Carl Munson. For your invaluable skills and support with regard to www.thetrueyoudiet.com.

Debbie Vandepeer – my assistant. For your brilliant organizational abilities, and for being such a hilarious and irreverent friend for two decades.

Barbara Vesey – my editor. For providing the original manuscript with some much-needed spit and polish.

Sandra Gomes. For being such a very special person, and for only very occasionally grumbling about my general absence while writing this book!

Contents

Introduction

Diet is a hot topic these days. Interest in this area has, to a large degree, been fuelled by the burgeoning rates of ills such as obesity and diabetes seen not just in adults, but in children too. No wonder, then, that there has been increasing emphasis on the need to shape ourselves up by shaping up what we put into our mouths.

Yet, while there is very little disagreement that we need to make collective changes to our diet, there is not as much agreement about what these changes should be.

If you take any interest in diet at all, you will no doubt be aware of just how often nutritional advice seems to flick-flack between concepts that can be contradictory, conflicting and, quite frankly, downright confusing. Perhaps the most obvious example of this concerns the recommendations given to us about how much fat and carbohydrate there should be in our diet.

The backbone of official nutritional advice over the last few decades has been that we should consume a low-fat diet, rich in starchy staples such as bread, potatoes, rice, pasta and breakfast cereals. Standard recommendations tell us to consume at least six portions of such foods each day if we want to shrink our waistlines as well as curb our risk of conditions such as heart disease and diabetes. On the other hand, some claim that the starchy carbs are actually the true culprits in the rapidly rising rates of conditions such as obesity and diabetes. Proponents of this approach tell us to give these foods a wide berth, and that there's nothing to be feared in the fats we are traditionally warned off.

And the confusion about what healthy eating means doesn't end there. Others espouse the virtues of, say, the 'correct' combining of foods, a diet based on raw foods, or eating according to one's blood group. There is undoubtedly a bewildering array of dietary concepts and theories out there, so it's no surprise that some of us can end up not knowing *who* or *what* to believe.

One thing that no doubt contributes to the uncertainty about a healthy diet is that every regime will have its success stories and supporters. Practically *any* diet, including those that look diametrically opposed, will work for some individuals, of course. However, having worked with literally thousands of individuals in clinical practice over the years, I know that every diet has its fair share of failures, too. Maybe you know this from your own personal experience. Have you, for instance, ever embarked optimistically and enthusiastically on a diet that has come highly recommended, only to find that it simply didn't work for *you*? Or maybe you got some initial benefit with a particular approach, only for this to peter out all too soon. Perhaps you found a diet that others claimed to find energizing and slimming actually caused you to *gain* weight and feel sluggish?

Experiences such as these, which I have witnessed countless times in both my professional and personal life, have convinced me of one simple truth: there is no one single healthy diet.

I have seen, for instance, individuals thrive on a vegetarian or vegan diet, and find foods such as fruits, vegetables, beans and lentils to be satisfying and enlivening. Often, these individuals can find eating a fat-rich diet causes them to feel 'heavy' immediately after a meal and prone to weight gain in the long term. However, for other individuals, a diet relatively devoid of fat may simply fail to really satisfy their appetite, and as a result can find themselves on an almost constant quest for food. For these individuals, eating 'heavier', fatty foods such as red meat and buttered vegetables will often actually speed weight loss and improve their energy levels and even mood.

Such variation in people's responses to diet may seem anecdotal, but is supported by scientific data, too. There's plenty of evidence out there that while a specific diet may work for some, it won't work for others. In one study published in the *Annals of Internal Medicine* the effects of a low-carbo-hydrate (high-fat) and a low-fat (high-carbohydrate) diet were assessed.[1] On the low-carb regime, some individuals lost in excess of 20kg, while others lost virtually nothing. In stark contrast to this, some participants lost consid-erable quantities of weight on the low-fat diet – but again, for others it was, to all intents and purposes, useless.

It really does seem that one person's meat can be another's poison.

So, what might account for the variability in the effects diets seem to have? The answer is to be found in something known as 'biochemical individuality'. Just as our external characteristics can vary enormously, so can our internal chemistry, too. The details of our physiological and biochemical workings determine, essentially, a food's suitability for our consumption. For instance, while some people have the capacity to digest the milk sugar lactose, others have not. Those lacking the lactose-digesting enzyme (known as lactase) in their digestive tracts will tend to ferment lactose in the gut, which can lead to symptoms such as bloating, flatulence and diarrhoea. Those individuals whose digestive tracts are capable of producing lactase, however, have no such problems with lactose.

Another example of biochemical individuality concerns the metabolism of alcohol. Normally, alcohol is broken down in the liver through the action of an enzyme known as 'alcohol dehydrogenase'. In some individuals, this enzyme is lacking, and this can cause affected individuals to be very sensitive to alcohol and quickly suffer from symptoms such as weakness, flushing of the face, and nausea if they drink it.

These examples of biochemical individuality have been known of for decades and are well enshrined in conventional medical teachings. However, more recently there has been growing awareness in the scientific community that our biochemical individuality can also determine our requirements for other dietary elements, including what are known as the major 'macronutrients' such as carbohydrate and fat. As we will explore in this book, scientific evidence shows that our ability to handle macronutrients varies considerably from person to person. This, as we shall see, has profound implications when it comes to determining our own ideal diet.

One might ask *why* it is that there is such apparent variation in our nutritional requirements. The explanation resides in our ancient past. Through the process of evolution, our species has changed and adapted to its environment in a way that has ensured its survival. For example, our ancestors evolving in sun-drenched parts would have benefited from darker skin tones. However, ancestors hailing from colder climes would not have had so much use for dark skin. In fact, for these individuals dark skin would have put them at a distinct disadvantage, because it reduces the body's ability to manufacture the health-giving nutrient vitamin D from sunlight. In this way, our external environment has helped shape the external appearance of our species.

The same is true of our internal characteristics, too. Individuals who were best suited to foods available at a given time and place would have been most likely to survive to pass these genes on to the next generation. In this way, our species became adapted to 'primal' foods that were commonly found in our evolutionary diet, such as meat, fish, fruit, vegetables and nuts. However, as we shall discover in the first chapter of this book (What On Earth Did We Eat?), there really was no such thing as a single 'primal diet'. Those of our ancestors who evolved in warm climates with a lot of vegetation, for instance, are likely to have eaten and become adapted to a diet rich in plant foods such as fruits and vegetables. On the other hand, animal foods such as meat and fish are likely to have been a near necessity for the survival of those who evolved in colder climes.

Again, through evolutionary adaptation our internal characteristics may reflect our ancestral eating habits. In this way, we might imagine that deep down in our genetic code, some of us are essentially 'hunters', and will therefore do best on a diet that contains relatively high-protein and fat-rich foods such as meat. Others, though, are genetically 'gatherers', and will suit a more plant-based diet with less in the way of fat in it. Still others – the 'hunter-gatherers' – will achieve optimal health through a diet somewhere between these two extremes.

The True You Diet gives you the tools to enable you to discover which of these three main 'types' you are. Nutritional science and practice show that your type can be determined by specific clues given by the body itself. Our appetite for foods and response to them, as well as other factors including certain physical and mental characteristics, can be used to determine your ideal diet. There is nothing new in this, of course: the practice of 'reading' the body in order to determine someone's specific nutritional needs has been employed in Ayurveda (Indian medicine) and other ancient forms of healing for literally thousands of years. In *The True You Diet* we use science to explain what traditional practitioners have known for a very long time indeed.

The True You Diet will not only reveal the type of diet that is right for you, but will also provide you with plenty of practical tips and recipes to allow you to incorporate your ideal diet into your life. By feeding your body the fuel best suited to it, you stand the very best chance of attaining the healthy weight and vibrant well-being that might, up until now, have seemed beyond your grasp.

There are, of course, other reasons why diets 'fail', including a tendency for some to take an 'all or nothing' approach to healthy eating. Not uncommonly, individuals can find themselves repeatedly getting on and off dietary regimes. While some short-term success may be had, there's often a trend towards gradually increasing weight and deterioration in well-being. The common causes of this phenomenon, and how to combat them successfully in the long term, are covered in depth in the final chapter of this book (Looking to the Future).

But before we can look to the future, we need to look back at our past. It is in our evolutionary history that we are most likely to find the diet and foods we are best adapted to and that are best for us. It may seem a little far-fetched to suggest that our ideal diet in the 21st century may be determined by what our ancestors were eating a million or more years ago. But we need to understand that our capacity to adapt to our changing environment, including our diet, relates to evolution, which is a very slow process indeed. Genetically, we are more than 99.9 per cent the same as our ancestors from 10,000 years ago, when our diet began to transform in fundamental ways. The first two chapters of this book (What on Earth Did We Eat? and Where Did It All Go Wrong?) chart the evidence for the diet that sustained us for some 2½ million years and the health issues that arose as soon as we began to stray from it. The third chapter of this book (All Change) describes the major adjustments we have seen in our diet in recent times, and takes a look at just how very different this is from our ancient diet. We shall see that foods introduced into our diet quite recently (in evolutionary terms) such as grains, refined sugar, dairy products, refined vegetable oils and industrially produced 'partially hydrogenated' fats now make up more than three-quarters of our diet.

In subsequent chapters, the scientific evidence for each of these foods is examined. In particular, we shall see what support there is for the 'healthy' properties of grains and dairy products, and explore what potential hazards these and other relative newcomers can pose for our health.

The True You Diet will also take a close look at the foods that made up our 'primal' diet. There is good evidence, for instance, that red meat has featured significantly in the human diet for pretty much all of our evolution, and we shall see that the scientific evidence reveals that this food and other 'forbidden' foodstuffs do not deserve their unhealthy reputation. Using the latest research, we will be appraising the pros and cons of not only meat, but other 'primal' foods such as fish, nuts, fruits and vegetables.

You may already be getting the impression that a lot of the information in this book is not in keeping with traditional nutritional 'wisdom' – and you'd be right. In the pages of this book you will find evidence which disproves a plethora of dietary 'facts'. These include the notions that dairy products are important for bone health, that margarine is 'healthier' than butter, that artificial sweeteners are a safe and effective weight-loss aid, and that starchy carbohydrates such as bread, potatoes, rice, pasta and breakfast cereals are somehow essential to good health. You will see, as you read this book, just how much dietary dogma has no foundation in science and is, to boot, contrary to common sense.

I have no doubt that some of the individuals who propagate these and other myths about nutrition are well-meaning, but simply do not realize just how misguided such notions are. But at the same time we need to be aware that much of the nutritional information that comes at us is tainted by commercial concerns. While this book is not intended as a political rant or polemic, we nonetheless need to be aware that food companies – and the organizations funded by them (including many bodies whose job it is to give 'official' pronouncements on what we should be eating) – have a habit of promoting concepts that are not in the interests of public health, but of *profit*. If you bear this in mind, you'll find it easier to reconcile how and why there can be such a yawning gap between what we are so often told and the truth.

Part of the role of this book is to provide you with the information that reveals what it *really* means to eat a healthy diet. This true understanding of the influence of foods on your health will help you to make changes to your diet with comfort and confidence. A thorough and deep understanding of diet and nutrition is an essential ingredient for achieving sustainable, lasting change and the myriad of health benefits that come with it.

Chapter 1 What On Earth Did We Eat?

A basic tenet of this book is that a truly healthy diet is one that is based on the foods that we've eaten for longest in terms of our evolution. With this in mind, let's take a trip back in time to explore our evolutionary path and the 'primal' diet we ate along the way.

Where Did We Come From?

In scientific circles it is generally accepted that the species we now call 'man' is a distant descendant of the great apes which include gorillas, orangutans and chimpanzees. Genetically, we humans are most closely related to chimpanzees and bonobos (also sometimes known as 'pygmy' or 'dwarf' chimpanzees). While there is some truth in the stereotypical image of chimps chomping on bananas, it is also true that this particular primate supplements its diet with animal foods such as meat (which they hunt for) and insects.[1,2] Another food that features in the chimpanzee diet is eggs. Add this to the fruit and vegetable matter chimpanzees eat, and what is clear is that the animal regarded as our original evolutionary ancestor is very much an omnivore.

It is generally accepted that the genetic line that finally gave rise to the ascent of man split off from our primate relatives some 6 million years ago.[3,4] The ancestors who made this genetic break formed an animal family known as the 'hominins' (formerly known as 'hominids'). The early hominins are believed to have spent much of their time in dry, bush-covered land,[5,6] and while, initially, the hominin diet almost certainly closely resembled that of the chimpanzee, there is evidence that by 3–4 million years ago our typical fare had seen significant change.

The record shows that the passage of time saw the development of smaller canine teeth (used to kill and eat prey), along with the development of larger molar teeth used for chewing. These dental developments suggest that foods requiring mastication, such as roots and tubers, assumed more prominence in the diet at this time.[7,8] This particular evolutionary step seems to have been important for the survival of our hominin ancestors by ensuring they had access to a steadier and more reliable supply of food throughout the year.

It is believed that our hominin ancestors transformed into our first truly 'human' ancestor, known as 'Homo habilis', about 2½ million years ago. These prototype humans sprung up in Africa, and had a brain about half the size of a modern-day human but substantially bigger than that of a chimpanzee. The enhanced brainpower enjoyed by Homo habilis allowed him to get to grips with some primitive stone tools. The gradually enlarging brain of our ancestors also, over time, allowed them to migrate from the relatively warm climes of Africa to other parts of the planet.

By about 1.7 million years ago our ancestors had made their way into colder, more temperate regions much further away from the equator. This time also saw the emergence of a taller, stockier, more upright ancestor known as 'Homo erectus'. The migration of this species to parts where there would have been a relative lack of edible vegetation would have made meat-eating a necessity for survival. Suitable prey for these early ancestors included mammoth and rhinoceros.[9] Also, patterns of wear and tear in the teeth suggest that the Homo erectus diet was rich in meat.[10] Other evidence for meat-eating comes from the finding of stone tools and bones scored by cut marks. The record indicates that the butchering of meat dates back some 2 million years.[11]

Another, less direct sign that meat had a significant place in our diet comes in the form of bony remains which show a gradual reduction in jaw size over this period of evolution. Scientists have generally interpreted this change to be a sign of increased consumption of meat (which is less fibrous than plant foods and therefore requires less chewing).

Some scientists have even suggested that the presence of meat in the diet actually helped propel our ancestors along the evolutionary road.[12] The reasoning behind this is that meat is rich in a fat known as 'arachidonic acid' (AA), an important building-block in brain tissue. Another important brain-builder is a fat known as 'docosahexaenoic acid' (DHA). DHA is a major constituent of fish oil, but is also found in brain tissue, as is AA. Bone marrow is another rich source of these brain-boosting fats. The relevance of this is that there is evidence that both animal brains and bone marrow are likely to have been scavenged foods that formed part of the Homo erectus diet. This idea is supported by the finding of stones dating back to the Homo erectus era which appear to be for the express purpose of breaking bones. The inclusion of bone marrow and brain in the diet may have been the critical factor in the brain enlargement that set our ancestors apart from their primate relations.

Big brains are generally an advantage in life, not least because they enhance the capacity to compete for food. Also, the improved brainpower gained at this time was almost certainly instrumental in the discovery and harnessing of fire, an estimated 0.5–1.5 million years ago. In addition to providing heat and protection, fire enabled our ancestors to cook foods, which would have improved the digestibility of other foodstuffs including roots and tubers.[13]

Around 900,000 years ago, the Earth experienced considerable cooling, and this seems to have made Homo erectus even more dependent on hunting for survival.[14] Subsequent to this, Homo erectus remains from China dating back some 400,000 years provide evidence of an omnivorous diet consisting of a variety of foods including mammals, reptiles, birds, eggs, fruit and tubers.[15]

From about this time on, evolution propelled the emergence of the immediate forerunners of our own species, in the form of what is known as 'Archaeic Homo sapiens'. Around 140,000–110,000 years ago, 'Homo sapiens' proper, characterized by an anatomy resembling that of modern humans, first made an appearance.

The discovery from this era of stone tools that look like they were used for hunting and butchering provides good evidence of widespread meat-eating. From about 40,000 years ago, there appears to have been a sudden explosion in the use of weapons and tools. This is why this period in ancient history is often referred to as the 'Stone Age'. Some have argued that the archaeological findings have skewed our beliefs about what constituted our diet at this time, on the basis that bone and tool artefacts persist long after plant matter in our diet might have evaporated.

Fortunately, modern science comes to the rescue here, as chemical analysis of bone and tooth enamel allows measurement of elements such as carbon and nitrogen which inform us about the likely protein content of the diet, and whether this protein was from an animal or plant source.[16–18]

Analysis of humans dating back some 30,000–13,000 years ago indicates a diet very rich in animal protein. Chemical analysis of tooth enamel also allows assessment, not just of the likely levels of protein in the diet, but of carbohydrates and fats, too.[19] It has been found that our quite recent ancestors ate protein and fats derived from fish and seafood, as well as land-dwelling animals. This perhaps comes as no surprise when we consider that between about 40,000 and 10,000 years ago our planet experienced a considerable drop in temperature (commonly referred to as the 'Ice Age') that would have necessitated our ancestors finding their food not just on land, but in lakes, rivers and the sea as well.

The end of the Ice Age saw a period of global warming that allowed our ancestors to broaden their diet. It was around this time, some 10,000 years ago, that agriculture first began. This enabled humans to establish a more stable supply of food in the form of plant foods, including grains.[20,21] The keeping and rearing of animals, and therefore the consumption of dairy products, appears to have come about a further 5,000 years later.

What is clear is that up until very recently in our evolutionary history, our diet was made up of natural foods that were both hunted and gathered, hence the reason why, prior to the development of agriculture and farming, we were described as 'hunter-gatherers'. However, it is highly likely that what constituted a hunter-gatherer's diet would have varied considerably depending on food availability. Some of our ancestors hailing from colder climes, for instance, would have eaten a diet rich in meat and perhaps fish, and are therefore better classified as 'hunters'. And those of our ancestors who evolved in habitats where vegetation made up much more of the diet are perhaps better described as 'gatherers'. Others, of course, will fall somewhere in between these extremes, and can therefore be best regarded as genuine hunter-gatherers. We shall explore the relevance of these basic types of ancestor to modern humans later in this book.

While there was no single 'primal diet', one thing for sure is that certain foods now commonplace in modern-day diets, such as grains and dairy products, are relative nutritional newcomers in the context of our entire evolution. In the next chapter (Where Did It All Go Wrong?) we will examine the potential consequences of introducing these and other, even more novel foods to our diet.

However, first we're going to further dissect the details of the hunter-gatherer diet. We can do this because not all of our ancestors took the agricultural route. Right up to the modern age, so-called hunter-gatherer populations still roamed many parts of the world. The diets of these populations are thought to reflect, to a large degree, the diet our ancestors ate prior to the agricultural age. Therefore, looking at the diets of the recent hunter-gatherers provides another useful window into our ancestral diet.

To date, the most comprehensive analysis of the make-up of hunter-gatherer diets was published in 2000 in the *American Journal of Clinical Nutrition*.[22] This review entailed an analysis of diets detailed in what is known as the *Ethnographic Atlas*. In this book, scientists and anthropologists have charted, amongst other things, the eating habits of dozens of modern hunter-gatherer populations from around the world. The Table on this page summarizes the findings of this analysis. This summary differentiates populations according to type of environment, and provides for each one the percentage of calories that come from gathered foods (such as fruits, vegetables, nuts and seeds), hunted foods (meat), and seafood and fish.

The most notable findings of this piece of research are:

Table 1.1

Environment	Dependence on gathered plant foods %	Dependence on hunted animal foods %	Dependence on fished animal foods %
Tundra, northern areas	6–15	36–45	46–55
Northern coniferous forest	16–25	26–35	46–55
Temperate forest, mostly mountainous	36–45	16–25	36–45
Desert grasses and shrubs	46–55	36–45	6–15
Temperate grassland	26–35	56–65	6–15
Subtropical bush	36–45	26–35	26–35
Subtropical rain forest	36–45	46–55	6–15
Tropical grassland	46–55	26–35	16–25
Monsoon forest	36–45	26–35	26–35
Tropical rain forest	26–35	26–35	36–45

- most (73%) of the populations studied derived more than 50% of their diets from animal foods.

- in contrast, only 13.5% of populations studied derived more than 50% of their diets from plant foods.

- of 229 hunter-gatherer populations, 58% obtained two-thirds or more of their diet from animal foods.

- in contrast, only 4% of societies obtained two-thirds or more of their diet from plant foods.

- 20% of hunter-gatherer populations were found to be highly or solely dependent on fished and hunted animal foods.

- in contrast, no hunter-gatherer population was found to be largely or entirely dependent on gathered plant foods.

Not surprisingly, reliance on animal foods is found to increase with increasing latitude. Basically, the further away from the equator and the colder it gets, the more a population will rely on animal foods to survive.

This evidence further strengthens the notion that our ancient diet was omnivorous, and contained varying amounts of animal and plant foods depending on environment, climate and season. Whatever the details of the 'primal' diet happen to be, what we know for sure is that for practically all of our time on this planet we ate nothing but natural, unprocessed foods such as meat, fish, seafood, fruits, vegetables and nuts. In theory, it is these foods that we are best adapted to from an evolutionary perspective. In the next chapter, we're going to be examining the evidence for this notion by seeing what happens when we stray too far, nutritionally speaking, from our primal path.

The Bottom Line

- The most appropriate diet for modern-day humans is one based on the foods we have become adapted to through the process of evolution.

- The evidence suggests we have evolved from chimpanzees, which are omnivorous in nature.

- Evidence from archaeological remains and the chemical analyses of bones and teeth reveal meat-eating was almost certainly a feature of our diet for the whole of our evolution.

- The migration of our ancestors and climatic change would have made meat-eating a necessity for survival at certain times.

- Analysis of the diets of modern 'hunter-gatherer' populations reveal generally high reliance on animal foods, particularly for those living in cold climates.

- There was no single 'primal' diet; the relative amounts of animal and plant foods varied considerably according to climate and food availability.

- It is only relatively recently (in terms of our evolution) that our species first ate foods that are now staples in the modern-day diet, such as grains and dairy products.

Chapter 2 **Where Did It All Go Wrong?**

In the last chapter we explored our ancient diet and discovered that, until relatively recently, the foods we subsisted on were those found naturally in nature, such as meat, fish, fruits, vegetables and nuts. From about 10,000 years ago, though, many of our ancestors chose to turn their back on their 'hunter-gatherer' heritage, and began instead to settle down, grow their own foods and, later on, to herd animals.[1] On the face of it, this development seems to have been a major boon for our species, in that it would have helped ensure a more reliable supply of food. This era, sometimes referred to as the 'Neolithic revolution', also led to a rapid increase in population numbers, and a way of life that finally culminated in what we know today as 'civilization'.

This turning point in our way of life is often hailed as a huge step forward for our species. But is it possible that it turned out to be a big step back in terms of our well-being? Bearing in mind the slow pace of genetic adaptation and evolution, could the dietary changes we have seen in the last few thousand years have ushered in a dietary dark age which has ultimately proved disastrous for our health?

What Bones and Teeth Tell Us About Our Ancient Health

While we do not have a detailed record of the state of the health of our ancient ancestors from thousands of years ago, we can nonetheless glean some valuable information about this by examining the remains of their bones and teeth. There is evidence, for instance, that the Neolithic age brought with it a significant deterioration in our dental health, with decay becoming much more prevalent at this time.[2]

Bones dating from this period also bear the scars of our move to grain-eating. The spread of corn-growing has been found to be associated with shorter stature in those of our ancestors who lived in a range of locations including North America,[3-6] Central America[7,8] and South America.[9] The fall in average height that came with the introduction of agriculture is in the order of 4–6 inches (10–15cm).[10]

There are several reasons why the adoption of grain-eating might have led to a deterioration in bone health and some shrinking in size. For example, there is evidence that the consumption of fruits and vegetables can help assist bone-building by making the body's internal environment less acidic, thus reducing the risk that calcium is 'leached' from the bone. A move away from 'alkalinizing' fruits and vegetables towards grains, which tend to acidify the body, might therefore impair the formation of healthy bones. Many grains (such as wheat) also contain substances (such as phytates) that impair the absorption of calcium. And there is also evidence that wholegrain cereals interfere with the metabolism of vitamin D, which has important implications for bone health.[11] Other evidence relating to changes in the shape and size of skulls and pelvic bones that date back to this time suggest that children of this era were less well nourished than those that came before them. The evidence we have from the archaeological record shows that the advent of agriculture and our increasing appetite for grain brought with it a clear deterioration in our health.

Of course, we don't necessarily need to go back 10,000 years in time to see what happens when individuals discard their indigenous diet in favour of novel foods. In the last century alone there has been plenty of opportunity to compare the diets and health status of individuals eating traditional foods, with those eating the typically 'Western' fare most of us will be familiar with.

Perhaps the most detailed study of this kind ever undertaken was conducted by an American dentist by the name of Dr Weston Price in the early part of the 20th century. Dr Price noticed during his work that increasing numbers of his adult patients were suffering from chronic and degenerative diseases, and that his younger patients were becoming increasingly afflicted by dental issues including crooked teeth and cavities.

Curious about what could be causing what seemed to be such a rapid erosion in health, Dr Price set about seeking an explanation. Price had heard that individuals who were members of native cultures were generally in good health and free of the sort of health problems he was seeing in his patients in the US state of Ohio. Price made it his mission to see whether this was indeed true, and if so, what it was that seemed to account for the abundant health of these 'primitive' people.

Accompanied by his wife, Price embarked on a nine-year voyage of discovery in which the health of peoples who were relatively untouched by civilization was meticulously documented. In all, Price and his wife studied 14 cultures around the world, in places as diverse as the Swiss Alps, islands off the coast of Scotland, the Andes in Peru, Africa, the Polynesian islands, Australia, New Zealand, northern Canada and the Arctic Circle.

Price documented his observations in his seminal book entitled *Nutrition and Physical Degeneration* which was first published in 1939. In this book, Price presented detailed information about the diets of those he studied. There was, not surprisingly, quite a large degree of variation here, which depended on a number of factors including custom and food availability.

Eskimos, for instance, were found to eat a diet almost completely made up of animal foods such as fish, walrus and seal. Other populations accustomed to finding a lot of their food in the sea were the Maori of New Zealand and the South Sea islanders. Fish, shark, octopus and shellfish all took some place in the diet, which was also supplemented with foods such as pork, coconut and fruit.

On the other hand, hunter-gatherer populations in Northern Canada, the Florida Everglades, the Amazon and Australia consumed less fish and more in the way of meat. In addition, they were also found to consume grains, beans, tubers, vegetables and fruits when available. African cattle-keeping tribes like the Masai were found to subsist on a very animal food-based diet based on beef, raw milk and blood. The Dinkas of the Sudan, whom Price regarded to be the healthiest of all the African tribes he studied, ate a combination of fermented whole grains, fish, red meat, vegetables and fruit. The Bantu, on the other hand, considered by Price as the least hardy of the African tribes he studied, were primarily agriculturists. Their diet consisted mostly of beans, squash, corn, millet, vegetables and fruits, with only small amounts of milk and meat.

Swiss mountain villagers were found to consume a diet rich in unpasteurized and cultured dairy products (especially butter and cheese), along with rye bread. Beef formed a small part of their diet, and this was supplemented with bone broths, vegetables and berries. Gaelic fisher people of the Outer Hebrides ate no dairy products, but instead had their fill of cod and other sea foods, especially shellfish when in season. Oats were grown, and these formed an important part of their diet.

While there was wide variation in the diets Price studied, there were some factors that were common to all. None of the populations Price encountered were vegetarian, and every diet was made up of ostensibly natural, unprocessed foods. There was no sign of any of the common modern-day foodstuffs such as white flour, refined sugar, pasteurized and homogenized dairy products or refined vegetable oils. And notably, the diets consumed by the cultures Price studied contained nothing in the way of chemical preservatives, additives, colourings or sweeteners.

A dentist by trade, it's perhaps no surprise that Price focused quite a lot on the dental health of the individuals he studied. Tellingly, wherever he and his wife went, dental decay was found to be almost non-existent. Price was also struck by the straightness and whiteness of the teeth he examined – this despite the fact that the cultures he examined were not accustomed to the use of either toothbrushes or toothpaste. Price also noticed that, in addition to their healthy teeth and gums, the individuals he studied had robust health, despite the sometimes challenging living conditions they had to endure.

Price also had the opportunity to assess the health of colonialists found living close to the more 'primitive' populations he studied, as well as some individuals from those primitive societies who had opted to adopt more modern eating habits. In local colonialists, Price found much more evidence of disease such as dental decay and tuberculosis than found in the primitive societies. Price also found that the natives who had abandoned their traditional eating habits in favour of something more 'Westernized' suffered from ill-health and rotting teeth as a result.

To some of us it may seem bizarre that dietary change could lead so quickly to such an obvious deterioration in health. However, bearing in mind that our ideal diet is largely dictated by our genes, and the fact that these change *very slowly*, it becomes quite obvious that a major change in our diet is likely to bring, quite quickly, potentially disastrous consequences to our internal chemistry and health.

The evidence clearly shows that turning our backs on our primal diet can have perilous consequences for our health. In the next chapter we're going to explore just how different our modern-day diet is from that which sustained the evolution of our species for some 2½ million years.

So Why Are We Living Longer?

If a change from our indigenous diet to a more modern one is so damaging to our health, how is it that we're living longer now than ever before? Before Neolithic times, the average lifespan was estimated to be 35 years for men and 30 years for women.[12] That doesn't compare at all well with, say, the current life expectancies of about 75 and 80 for men and women respectively in England and Wales. However, our ancient ancestors were at the mercy of factors such as warfare, starvation, extreme climate and animal attack which are generally not so much of an issue now. Also, developments in medicine, hygiene and sanitation have been massively instrumental in reducing the risk of death due to, say, childbirth and infectious disease. At the same time, the evidence strongly suggests that a departure from our natural diet brings with it an increased risk of ill-health. The logical conclusion to be drawn from these facts is that our increased life expectancy has not been because of recent changes in our diet, but *in spite* of them.

The Bottom Line

- The introduction of grains into the human diet some 10,000 years ago was accompanied by a decline in our height, and a deterioration in our dental health and general nutritional status.

- Evidence from the last century shows that populations eating a natural, unprocessed diet generally have very robust health and well-being, despite sometimes very challenging living conditions.

- Recent evidence also shows that our departure from an indigenous diet towards one containing 'Western' foods brings with it significant hazards for our health.

Chapter 3 **All Change**

Taking a look at the typical Western diet, it's difficult to see any real resemblance to the primal diet we evolved on. Prior to the Neolithic era, foods now commonplace in the diet, such as grains and dairy products, were simply not eaten. In very recent years we have seen the introduction of considerable quantities of refined sugar, refined vegetable oils and refined flour products which, again, simply did not pass our lips for the very great majority of our evolution.[1]

In this chapter we're going to be taking a long, hard look at the modern-day diet, and compare it to the diet we ate prior to the dawn of civilization. The major changes we have seen in the human diet since our hunter-gatherer days relate to our consumption of grains, refined sugar, dairy products, refined and processed vegetable oils, alcohol and salt. Here, we're going to look at each one of these foods to get an overall picture of how much our diet has really changed in recent times.

Grains

The growing and consumption of grains started only 10,000 years ago. It seems likely that, initially, grains were used to supplement the existing diet – mass agriculture for feeding of the masses did not occur overnight. Also, grains would have first been consumed in a minimally processed form. Things are very different now, of course. Grain-based foods such as bread, rice, pasta and breakfast cereals now account for about a third of the total calories we consume as a population.[2]

And it's not just the quantity of grain we are consuming that might have some relevance to our health, but its *quality*. While the grains we first consumed were minimally processed, the Industrial Revolution of the late 18th and early 19th century allowed the refining of grain on a scale never before known in our history. These processes not only can strip grain of much of what nutrients it contains naturally, but also tend to cause the grain to liberate the sugar it contains more quickly into the bloodstream. This is an issue we shall explore in more depth in the next chapter (Against the Grain).

Finally, the strains of certain grains, particularly wheat, can be quite different now to those that were first cultivated. This has important implications for our health, particularly with regard to an issue known as 'food intolerance'. This issue is also examined in the next chapter.

Refined Sugar

While sugar, say in fruit, has been in our diet for ever, the same cannot be said for so-called 'refined' sugar which is extracted from one food (such as sugar beet, sugar cane or corn) to then be *added* to another (such as a soft drink, fruit yoghurt, dessert or bar of chocolate). One critical difference here is that sugar found naturally in food (known as 'intrinsic' sugar) tends to liberate itself more slowly into the bloodstream than sugar that has been added to a food (known as 'extrinsic' sugar). As we shall see in the next chapter (Against the Grain), this has very important implications for health.

While the refining of sugar is thought to date back 2,500 years,[3] it was not until after the Industrial Revolution some 200 years ago that refined sugar consumption really took off. Refined sugar now accounts for about 13 per cent of total calories we consume.[4] The hazards of consuming refined sugar are discussed in Chapter 5 (Sweet and Sour).

Dairy Products

The first real evidence for the consumption of milk products comes from chemical analysis of pottery that dates back about 5,000 years ago.[5] As with grains, our intake of dairy products almost certainly started slowly. Now, dairy foods account for about 10 per cent of the total calories we consume.[6]

As with many grain-based foods, it's not just the quantity, but also the quality of dairy products that has changed. Pasteurization, for instance, is a very recent development that might have important consequences with regard to the health effects of dairy foods, particularly with regard to food sensitivity. The health effects of dairy products will be discussed in Chapter 6 (Slaying the Sacred Cow).

Refined and Industrially Processed Vegetable Oils

'Vegetable' oils have always been in the diet in certain fruits (e.g. olives and avocado), vegetables and nuts. The Industrial Revolution brought with it food-processing techniques that allowed the mass-production of oils. In this way, very recently we have begun to consume vegetable oils in quantities that far exceed those possible when we consume the whole foods from which these oils are obtained.

Official UK statistics do not allow us to know how much refined vegetable oil we consume, but it's likely to be in the same order of magnitude of that in the US, which currently stands at about 18 per cent of total calories consumed.

Another major development concerning vegetable oils is a process known as 'partial hydrogenation', which can be used to solidify oils as well as extend their shelf lives. Unfortunately, this process, which dates back only a century, can generate completely novel forms of fats, known as 'trans fatty acids', that were essentially absent from the diet we ate in pre-agricultural times. More information about these fats and the potential impact of eating them can be found in Chapter 7 (Oil Crisis).

Alcohol

The drinking of alcohol may be embedded in many cultures around the world, but the evidence suggests that this habit dates back around 7,000 years.[7] Currently, alcohol intake accounts for about 6.5 per cent of caloric consumption in men and 4 per cent in women.[8] Moderate alcohol consumption is often promoted as 'healthy', particularly with regard to the heart. We shall be examining the evidence regarding the health effects of alcohol in Chapter 10 (Fluid Thinking).

Salt

The earliest use of salt as a food additive is argued to have taken place in China some 8,000 years ago.[9] In all likelihood, though, primitive 'hunter-gatherer' societies added little or no salt to their food. Contrast this with modern-day intakes in the UK, which stand at an average of 11.0g per day for men and more than 8.0g per day for women.

Excessive salt intake can raise blood pressure – something which is generally believed to increase the risk of heart attacks and strokes. Put another way, cutting back on our salt consumption could reduce the risk of these conditions. In one study, researchers from the Blood Pressure Unit at St George's Hospital in London in the UK assessed data from 29 trials examining the effect of salt reduction on blood pressure.[10] The data from this review suggest that if we in the UK halved our salt consumption, we would see meaningful reductions in blood pressure, and – for those suffering with high blood pressure – a 9 per cent reduction in deaths due to heart disease and a 14 per cent reduction in deaths due to stroke.

About 10 per cent of the salt consumed now is found naturally in foods. Another 10 per cent is added during cooking or at the table. This means that the vast majority of the salt we consume comes in processed foods where additional salt has been added during their production.

For those keen to reduce their salt intake, foods worth avoiding include savoury snacks, tinned vegetables, cheese and processed meats such as bacon, ham, sausages and beefburgers, as well as bread and breakfast cereals (cornflakes, for instance, contain the same salt concentration as sea water).

That Was Then, This Is Now

So, what do these changes look like when we put them all together and compare them to our diet of old? Well, prior to some 10,000 years ago, our diet was essentially devoid of grains, dairy products, refined sugar, refined vegetable oils, partially hydrogenated fats or alcohol.

Now these foods make up more than 75 per cent of the calories we consume.

Can We Cope?

There is no doubt that, as a species, we have *some* capacity to adapt to dietary changes. One example of this concerns the digestion of the milk sugar lactose, mentioned in the Introduction to this book. Lactose is broken down in the gut by an enzyme known as lactase. Infant humans are born with the ability to secrete lactase in order for them to be able to digest the lactose in their mother's milk. However, 70 per cent of the world's population will eventually lose the ability to produce lactase, and become what is known as 'lactose intolerant'. Individuals with lactose intolerance will typically find that consuming lactose can lead to digestive symptoms such as diarrhoea and wind.

It is well known that the capacity to digest lactose is quite strongly tied to race. Afro-Caribbeans and Asians, for instance, are generally poor digesters of lactose. Caucasians, on the other hand, are usually able to digest lactose.

It has been suggested that developing the ability to digest lactose was an advantage to races evolving in cold climates, as it allowed them to use milk as a ready form of food.[11] This supports the idea that even in our relatively recent past there has been some evolutionary adaptation to our diet.

However, there are limits. It needs to be borne in mind that our capacity to adapt to our changing diet is limited by evolution, which is generally a very slow process indeed. So, while we may be able to get away with some dietary change, having more than three-quarters of our diet come from quite new foods is very likely to have exceeded our capacity to cope.

In later chapters we shall be looking in some depth at the likely health effects these relatively novel foods have on health. However, before we dive into the detail, we're going to consider how recent dietary adjustments have affected our intake of broad nutritional elements such as carbohydrate, protein and fat.

You may remember that in the first chapter we explored the make-up of our evolutionary diet by looking at the archaeological remains, and also through analysis of primitive hunter-gatherer diets.[12] The Table below compares the relative amounts of carbohydrate, protein and fat in hunter-gatherer diets with those in the typical UK diet:

Table 3.1

Food component	'Hunter-gatherer' diet – percentage of total calories	Typical UK diet – percentage of total calories
Carbohydrate	22–40	46
Protein	19–35	16
Fat	28–58	33

We can see from this Table that, compared to our more primitive diet, we are consuming:

• significantly more carbohydrate

• significantly less protein

• generally less fat

The evidence shows that our diet has undergone a wholesale transformation over a relatively short period in our evolution. Let's now look in more depth at the likely effects associated with our rapidly changing diet, starting with the foodstuff we are often encouraged to base our diet on – grain.

The Bottom Line

• The pre-agricultural diet was almost exclusively made up of foods such as meat, fish, shellfish, eggs, nuts, fruit and vegetables.

• Grains were first introduced into the human diet some 10,000 years ago, followed by dairy products about 5,000 years ago.

• Much more recent additions to the diet include refined sugar, refined vegetable oils and industrially produced fats known as partially hydrogenated fats and trans fatty acids.

• 'New' foods such as these now make up more than three-quarters of the modern-day diet.

• Compared to more primitive, indigenous diets, we now consume significantly more carbohydrate and less protein, and generally less fat.

Chapter 4 **Against the Grain**

Grain-based foods such as bread, rice, pasta and breakfast cereals are staples in the Western diet, and are often promoted on account of the fact they provide valuable energy for the body whilst being naturally low in fat. Wholegrains such as wholemeal bread, certain breakfast cereals and brown rice, we are told, have the added advantage of being rich in fibre and essential nutrients. No wonder, then, that doctors, dieticians and health agencies tell us that each one of us should consume six or more portions of these starchy carbs each day, and that such fare should form the cornerstone of our diets.

However, the fact that grains, particularly refined ones, are a relatively recent addition to the diet means that we might question the notion of using them as the basis of our diet. If primal nutritional theory holds true, then grain-based foods might not be the superfoods they're cracked up to be. So are grains really the staff of life?

From Starch into Sugar

Central to our assessment of the effect grain-based foods have on health is an understanding of the effect they have on the body's biochemistry and physiology. Grains are primarily composed of starch, which itself is comprised of chains of sugar molecules. Once a starchy food is eaten it must be broken down through digestion into sugar before it can be absorbed through the gut wall and into the bloodstream. This means that whether we eat sugar, starch, or a combination of both, blood-sugar levels will rise.

As levels of sugar in the bloodstream start to climb, the body brings into play mechanisms that are designed to keep them from rising too high. Key to this process is the hormone insulin, which is secreted by an organ called the pancreas.

One of insulin's chief effects is to help the transport of sugar from the bloodstream into the body's cells. Without any insulin, sugar levels in the bloodstream rise uncontrollably, with potentially fatal consequences.

However, while insulin is essential to life, you can always get too much of a good thing. Should blood-sugar levels in the body rise considerably, then the surges of insulin that may result can cause blood-sugar levels to nose-dive some time (generally 2–4 hours) later. As we shall see later on in this chapter, many modern starch-based foods give up their sugar very readily, and consequently have considerable potential to induce gluts of insulin – and the episodes of low blood sugar that tend to follow.

Some of the most common symptoms of lower-than-normal blood-sugar levels (the medical term for which is 'hypoglycaemia') include:

- **Fatigue**
  Sugar provides ready fuel for the body, and if the level of sugar in the blood drops, fatigue is almost inevitable. Individuals with blood-sugar imbalance tend to experience peaks and troughs of energy as a result of the rise and fall in blood-sugar levels.

- **The mid-afternoon slump**
  The rise in blood sugar that follows lunch can trigger a rush of insulin that can lead to low blood sugar later on. Classically, this is responsible for the slump in energy many individuals experience in the mid-late afternoon (usually 3.30–5.00 p.m.).

- **Poor concentration, low mood or irritability**
  Although the brain makes up only about 2 per cent of our weight, at rest it uses roughly half the sugar circulating in our bloodstream. Blood-sugar imbalance quite commonly causes problems with poor concentration, depression, irritability and mood swings.

- **Waking in the night**
  When blood-sugar levels drop during the night, the body may attempt to correct this by secreting hormones which stimulate the internal fuelling of the system through, for instance, the release of sugar from the liver. The hormones the body uses to liberate fuel in this way are 'stress' hormones such as adrenaline and cortisol. This is a common

cause of waking in the night, and can often make it difficult to get back to sleep again.

- **Food cravings**

  Another common symptom of hypoglycaemia is food cravings. When blood-sugar levels drop to sub-normal levels, it's natural for our body to desire foods it knows will restore the blood-sugar level quickly. This commonly manifests as cravings for sweet foodstuffs such as chocolate, biscuits or sugary drinks.

Other Hazards of Insulin Excess

Driving blood-sugar to sub-normal levels is not the only effect that an excess of insulin has in the body. Besides the impact on blood-sugar balance, high levels of insulin pose other hazards for health. Insulin, to begin with, has the capacity to stimulate the production of fat in the body through the activation of an enzyme known as 'acetyl CoA carboxylase'. Insulin also has the ability to inhibit fat breakdown by suppressing the activity of an enzyme called 'lipase'.

What these effects can add up to is added weight. Any fatty accumulation that results from excesses of insulin tends to congregate around the midriff. You and I may know that as an additional roll or two, or full-blown 'spare tyre', but in medicine the term given to this form of excess baggage is 'abdominal obesity'.

Over the last decade or so, doctors and scientists have given increasing attention to abdominal obesity, partly because this particular type of weight distribution is strongly linked with an increased risk of major ills including Type 2 diabetes and heart disease. The term 'metabolic syndrome' (also sometimes referred to as 'syndrome X') has been coined to describe the problems associated with insulin excess. While the exact definition of this condition varies a bit, there is general acceptance that its diagnosis depends on the presence of abdominal obesity accompanied by two or more other common features associated with the condition.

- **Abdominal Obesity**

  For the purposes of diagnosing metabolic syndrome, abdominal obesity is generally defined as a waist size of 94cm (37 inches) or more for men and 80cm (31.5 inches) or more for women.

Another way of assessing the degree of abdominal obesity is by dividing the waist circumference by the circumference of the hips at their widest point. Higher 'waist-to-hip ratios' are associated with an increased risk of heart disease and diabetes.

The other features often used to establish the diagnosis of metabolic syndrome are:

- **Raised levels of blood fats known as 'triglycerides'**
  Triglycerides are one type of fat that can circulate in the bloodstream. Triglyceride levels of more than 1.7 mmol/l are generally regarded as elevated when metabolic syndrome is being considered.

- **Reduced levels of 'healthy' high-density lipoprotein (HDL) cholesterol**
  HDL is a particular form of cholesterol which is associated with a *reduced* risk of conditions such as heart disease and stroke. Levels of 0.9 mmol/l or less are generally regarded as relevant when metabolic syndrome is being considered.

- **Raised blood pressure**
  High blood pressure is believed to be a risk factor for heart attack and stroke. A systolic pressure of more than 130 mmHg and/or diastolic pressure of more than 85 mmHg is generally regarded as significant when metabolic syndrome is being considered.

- **Raised fasting blood-glucose level or previously diagnosed Type 2 diabetes**
  Type 2 diabetes is the most common form of diabetes, a common feature of which is an inability of insulin to function normally in the body – sometimes termed 'insulin resistance'. A fasting blood-sugar level of more than 5.6 mmol/l is generally regarded as significant when metabolic syndrome is being considered.

Metabolic syndrome and the insulin excess that tends to accompany it have been strongly linked with an increased risk of heart disease. The syndrome also appears to have associations with a wide variety of modern-day ills including short-sightedness, acne, gout, polycystic ovary syndrome[1] and an increased risk of certain cancers, including those of the breast, colon and prostate.

All this means that fluctuations in blood-sugar levels and excesses of the hormone insulin have potentially dire consequences for our well-being, as well as our health prospects in the long term. We need to have this in mind as we now go on to examine the effect that grains – the focus of this chapter – have on these critically important physiological processes.

Grains and Biochemical Balance in the Body

Nutritional 'wisdom' for a long time dictated that grains and other foods rich in 'complex carbohydrate', such as potatoes, give a healthy, tempered release of sugar into the bloodstream. This belief was based on the fact that the starch they contain has to be broken down into sugar prior to absorption, and this obviously takes time. More than two decades ago, scientists began to put this theory to the test by actually measuring the blood-sugar responses of individuals fed foods and drinks rich in sugar and/or starch. Specifically, researchers measured the amount of sugar released into the bloodstream in the two-hour period right after ingestion of the foodstuff being tested.

The term given to this way of quantifying the sugar release from a foodstuff is the 'glycaemic index' or 'GI'. One way of gauging the extent to which foods raise blood-sugar levels is to compare this to the body's response to consuming glucose (obviously, a very fast releasing food indeed). In the world of the GI, glucose is assigned a GI value of 100, and all other foods are compared to it. Basically, the higher a food's GI, the more disruptive its effects on blood-sugar and insulin levels.

The Effects of Glycaemic Index on Health

Before we take a look at the GI values of some of the most commonly consumed carbs, let's first examine what effect a food's GI is likely to have on health.

GI and Appetite

One of the most important effects GI has within the body concerns its effect on appetite. Basically, the higher a food's GI, the less satisfying it tends to be. Of 20 studies published between 1977 and 1999, 16 showed that low-GI foods promoted the satisfaction derived from that meal and/or reduced subsequent hunger.[2] Overall, the results of the studies show that an increase in the GI by 50 per cent reduces the satisfaction it gives by about 50 per cent. This has obvious and profound implications for anyone wanting to curb a tendency to overeat.

GI and Fat Metabolism
Earlier in this chapter, we discussed how excesses of insulin can stall the body's fat-burning potential. In one study, a high-GI meal was found, compared to a low-GI meal, to bring about relatively lower levels of fat metabolism, and that this effect lasted for several hours.[3]

GI and Diabetes
In theory, a diet rich in high-GI foods may increase the risk of Type 2 diabetes. It can do this by increasing insulin levels and therefore the risk that the body will become resistant to the effects of this hormone in time. Also, a high demand for insulin can cause the pancreas, which secretes it, to become 'exhausted', which can lead to diabetes through a relative lack of insulin.

In one study of 84,000 women,[4] higher intakes of white bread and potatoes (both high-GI foods) were significantly associated with a higher risk of diabetes.

On the other hand, a lower-GI diet would be expected to help in the management of diabetes. Several studies of people with diabetes have found that blood-sugar control was significantly improved when subjects consumed lower-GI diets.[5-12]

So, in short, eating foods of high GI has been linked with adverse effects on health including weight gain and an increased risk of diabetes. And, in the shorter term, high-GI foods' ability to destabilize blood-sugar levels can lead to problems such as fatigue, mental lethargy, food cravings and an inability to sleep soundly throughout the night.

Let's now look at the GIs of commonly eaten carbohydrate-rich foods (see table 4.1).

While there is continuing debate about how GIs should be classified, my preference is to call GIs of 70 or more 'high', GIs of 50–69 inclusive 'medium', and GIs of 49 or less 'low'.

What is very revealing is that the starchy carbohydrates, originally believed to give a slow and sustained release of sugar, actually turn out to

Table 4.1 Glycaemic Indices of Commonly Eaten Carbohydrates[13]

Breads	GI
baguette	95
bagel – white	72
wheat bread – white	70
bread – wholemeal	71
rye bread – wholemeal	58
rye bread – pumpernickel	46
bread – spelt, wholemeal	63

Crackers	GI
rye crispbread	64
cream cracker	65
water cracker	71
rice cakes	78
corn chips	63
potato crisps	54
popcorn	72

Pasta, rice and related foods	GI
brown rice	55
basmati rice	58
rice – arborio (risotto rice)	69
rice – white	64
barley – pearl	25
pasta – corn	78
gnocchi	68
pasta – durum wheat	44
pasta – wholewheat	37
cous cous	65

Sweet foods	GI
digestive biscuits	59
croissant	67
crumpet	69
doughnut	76
muffin – bran	60
scone	92

	GI
shortbread	64
ice cream	61
low-fat yoghurt	27
Mars bar	65
muesli bar	65
Snickers bar	55
honey	55
sucrose (table sugar)	68

Beverages	GI
apple juice – unsweetened	40
cranberry juice	56
orange juice	50
Gatorade	78
tomato juice	38
Coca cola	53
Fanta	68
Lucozade	95

Breakfast cereals	GI
All-Bran	42
bran flakes	74
cornflakes	81
muesli	40–66
porridge – homemade	58
porridge – instant	66
Special K	54–84
Shredded wheat	75
Raisin bran	61

Fruit	GI
apple	38
apple – dried	29
banana	52
mango	51
grapes	46
kiwi fruit	53

Food	GI		Food	GI
cherries	22		kidney beans	28
peach	42		lentils – green	30
pear	38		lentils – red	26
pineapple	59		peas – dried then boiled	22
plum	39		peas – boiled	48
watermelon	72			
figs – dried	61		**Vegetables**	**GI**
apricots – dried	31		parsnips	97
sultanas	60		potato – baked	85
raisins	64		potato – boiled	50
prunes	29		potato – new	57
strawberries	40		chips (French fries)	75
			potato – mashed	74
Legumes (beans, lentils, peas)	**GI**		potato – instant mashed	85
baked beans	48		yam	37
black-eyed beans	42		carrots – raw	16
butter beans	31		carrots – cooked	58
chickpeas	28		pumpkin	75
hummus	6		beetroot	64

be quite disruptive to the body's biochemistry. Many of these starchy staples – for instance cornflakes, wholemeal bread, risotto rice, rice cakes and cous cous – have high GIs. Some starches release sugar even more quickly than table sugar (sucrose).

Look closely at the GI list and you will see that some fruits and vegetables, including beetroot, pineapple and watermelon, have high-ish GIs, too. Does that mean that these foods are equivalent to foods with similar GIs such as corn chips and Mars bars? Actually, while the GI is an important measure of the nutritional attribute of a food, it's not the sole arbiter of a food's suitability for our consumption. One other factor that needs consideration is the *amount* we eat of a food: foods with a relatively high GI will be most disruptive if we eat a lot of them. The eating of foods of high or medium GI matters less if we don't tend to consume too much of them at any one time.

Therefore, anyone who goes hungry all day only to come home and polish off a bowlful or two of pasta is likely to experience considerable disruption in blood-sugar and insulin levels. On the other hand, it's highly unlikely that anyone, even when famished in the evening, is going to find themselves gorging themselves on mounds of beetroot or pineapple. When eaten, such foods are usually consumed in very moderate amounts, and thus are unlikely to cause much in the way of imbalance in sugar and insulin levels. Also, foods such as beetroot and pineapple are quite water-rich, which limits the amount of carbohydrate they contain and therefore their capacity to disrupt the body's biochemistry.

These concepts have spawned the development of another measure of the effect of food in the body: the 'glycaemic load'. The glycaemic load (GL) of a food is essentially calculated by multiplying its GI by the amount of carbohydrate contained in a typical portion of food. Basically, a food's GL is thought to give a more realistic guide to the impact of that food on blood sugar and insulin balance than its GI alone. What follows is a table of the GI and GL values of commonly eaten carbohydrates.

As with the GI, there is some debate about where we should be placing the boundaries between 'high', 'medium' and 'low' GL foods. My preference is to regard a GL of 20 or more as 'high', and one of 10 or less as 'low'. Anywhere in between I regard as 'medium'.

Now, looking at both the GIs and GLs of commonly eaten carbohydrates, we see a different picture emerging to the one painted when we judge foods by GI alone. Many of the foods that have medium or high GIs turn out to have low GLs. Examples include kiwi fruit (GI 53/GL 6), pineapple (GI 59/GL 7), watermelon (GI 72/GL 4), cooked carrots (GI 58/GL 3) and beetroot (GI 64/GL 5). On the other hand, many of the grain-based foods with medium or high GI have relatively high GLs, too. Examples include bagel (GI 72/GL 25), white rice (GI 65/GL 23), rice cakes (GI 78/GL 17), cornflakes (GI 81/GL 21) and pasta (GI 44/GL 21).

So, it's not just the fast sugar-releasing nature of the grain-based foods that poses problems for the body, but the fact that they tend to be very carbohydrate-rich and eaten in quantity. Overall, we might expect that eating less of these foods could help reduce both blood-sugar and insulin levels in the body. Let us not forget, either, that foods of high GI tend not to satisfy the appetite as much as lower-GI foods. Put all this together, and it stands to reason that cutting down on high-GI/GL carbs should help us shed excess weight.

Table 4.2 Glycaemic Indices and Glycaemic Loads of Commonly Eaten Carbohydrates[17]

Food	GI	GL
Breads		
baguette	95	15
bagel – white	72	25
wheat bread – white	70	10
bread – wholemeal	71	9
rye bread – wholemeal	58	8
rye bread – pumpernickel	46	5
bread – spelt, wholemeal	63	12
Crackers		
rye crispbread	64	11
cream cracker	65	11
water cracker	71	13
rice cakes	78	17
corn chips	63	17
potato crisps	54	11
popcorn	72	8
Pasta, rice and related foods		
brown rice	55	18
basmati rice	58	22
rice – arborio (risotto rice)	69	36
rice – white	64	23
barley – pearl	25	11
pasta – corn	78	32
gnocchi	68	33
pasta – durum wheat	44	21
pasta – wholewheat	37	16
cous cous	65	23
Sweet foods		
digestive biscuits	59	10
croissant	67	17
crumpet	69	13
doughnut	76	17

Food	GI	GL
muffin – bran	60	15
scone	92	7
shortbread	64	10
ice cream	61	8
low-fat yoghurt	27	7
Mars bar	65	26
muesli bar	65	26
Snickers bar	55	19
honey	55	10
sucrose (table sugar)	68	7 (10g)
Beverages		
apple juice – unsweetened	40	12
cranberry juice	56	16
orange juice	50	13
Gatorade	78	12
tomato juice	38	4
Coca cola	53	14
Fanta	68	23
Lucozade	95	40
Breakfast cereals		
All-Bran	42	8
bran flakes	74	13
cornflakes	81	21
muesli	40–66	12
porridge – homemade	58	13
porridge – instant	66	17
Special K	54–84	11–20
Shredded wheat	75	15
Raisin bran	61	12
Fruit		
apple	38	6
apple – dried	29	10

Food	GI	GL	Food	GI	GL
banana	52	12	chickpeas	28	8
mango	51	8	hummus	6	0
grapes	46	8	kidney beans	28	7
kiwi fruit	53	6	lentils – green	30	5
cherries	22	3	lentils – red	26	5
peach	42	5	peas – dried then boiled	22	2
pear	38	4	peas – boiled	48	3
pineapple	59	7	**Vegetables**		
plum	39	5	parsnips	97	12
watermelon	72	4	potato – baked	85	26
figs – dried	61	16	potato – boiled	50	14
apricots – dried	31	9	potato – new	57	12
sultanas	60	25	chips (French fries)	75	22
raisins	64	28	potato – mashed	74	15
prunes	29	10	potato – instant mashed	85	17
strawberries	40	1	yam	37	13
Legumes (beans, lentils, peas)			carrots – raw	16	1
baked beans	48	7	carrots – cooked	58	3
black-eyed beans	42	13	pumpkin	75	3
butter beans	31	6	beetroot	64	5

So, Does Cutting Carbs Actually Help Weight Loss?

There are, therefore, several theoretical reasons why low-carb diets may help weight loss, but do they perform in practice? The effects of low-GI or -GL diets on weight have been tested in several studies. In one, obese females consumed one of two calorie-restricted diets for 12 weeks.[18] Compared to those eating a high-GI diet, those consuming lower-GI food saw greater weight loss (7.4 compared with 4.5kg). In another study, a low-GI diet was compared to a conventional reduced-fat diet.[19] This study, like the last one, found a lower-GI diet was more effective in terms of weight loss. Another study, this time in pregnant women, found that those eating a high-GI diet gained substantially more weight compared to women eating a low-GI diet (19.7 compared with 11.8kg).[20]

The effects of several lower- and higher-carbohydrate diets were compared in a review published in the *Journal of the American Medical Association*. Overall, lower carbohydrate diets were found to bring about a weight loss of 12.4kg, compared with just 3.4kg on higher-carbohydrate regimes.[21] This review appears to provide compelling evidence for the potential effectiveness of carbohydrate restriction in weight loss.

Other research has focused on the relative merits of low-carb eating compared to the traditionally recommended approach to weight loss – the low-fat diet. To date, four well-designed trials have been performed which have pitted low-carbohydrate diets against low-fat diets over the medium-long term to assess their relative effects on weight.[22-5] All four studies found that weight loss after six months was 4 to 6kg greater in the low-carbohydrate group than in the low-fat group. Two of the studies lasted for a year.[26,27] At this point, the differences in weight loss had narrowed to 2kg and were no longer statistically significant.

It is worth bearing in mind that the diets tested were actually *very* low in carbohydrate, and there is considerable doubt about how sustainable this sort of eating is. In one study[28] compliance was monitored, and it turned out that most participants did not cut their carb consumption to the level they were asked to. In the other study[29] there was no checking of compliance at all. In other words, it is just not known whether the study participants restricted carbohydrate in the way or to the extent they were instructed to. Considering these deficiencies, these two studies cannot be used to judge the relative merits of carbohydrate or fat restriction in the long term.

In Chapter 8 (Lean Times) we will go on to see that low-fat diets have been shown to be thoroughly ineffective for the purposes of weight loss in the long term. Against this, let's not forget that lower-carb eating has been proven to bring far more in the way of weight loss than diets higher in carb.[30]

Is Extreme Carb Restriction Healthy or Necessary?

Low-carb diets have been brought to the public's attention largely through the popularity of diets such as the 'Atkins Diet' which, in their initial stages at least, are very low in carbohydrate indeed. Such extreme carbohydrate restriction can often get results. However, I have my reservations about how healthy these diets are, particularly in the long term. To my mind, there is too much restriction of relatively healthy carbohydrate sources such as fruits, vegetables, beans and lentils. Also, some of the advocated foods on such diets may be low in carb, but that does not make them automatically healthy. Hunks of cheese, artificially sweetened soft drinks and snack bars chock full of highly processed soya spring to mind.

The good news is that extreme carbohydrate restriction is simply unnecessary for effective weight loss anyway. In one study, a diet in which only 5 per cent of calories were contributed by carbohydrate (a very low carbohydrate diet) was pitted against one in which about 40 per cent of calories were contributed by carbohydrate.[31] Over six weeks, individuals in both groups on average lost about the same amount of weight (about 7kg). However, those on the less restrictive diet felt more energized and exhibited biochemical evidence of lower levels of inflammation in their bodies. Moderate, as opposed to extreme, carbohydrate restriction can help ensure sustainable weight loss, and is likely to be healthier, too.

Cutting Carbs – Is It Safe?

Despite their potential for effective weight loss, health professionals often view low-carb diets in a dim light. All the so-called 'saturated' animal fat that can come as part and parcel of such diets generally makes doctors and dieticians nervous about the effect this will have on health, particularly with regard to heart disease. As we shall see in Chapter 8 (Lean Times), the evidence shows that saturated fat is not a potent factor in heart disease at all. If we're going to point to any brand of fat in the diet as a factor in heart disease, it seems we should look to the industrially produced partially hydrogenated and 'trans' fats often found in foods such as biscuits, crackers, muffins and margarine. This is discussed in more detail in Chapter 7 (Oil Crisis).

The fatty foods that often feature in a low-carb diet are also often vilified on account of their cholesterol content. While there is some potential for low-carb diets to raise cholesterol levels in certain individuals, we shall see in Chapter 8 (Lean Times) that this is likely to make little or no difference to health. It should also be borne in mind that low-carb diets have been shown to have the capacity to lower levels of triglycerides and raise levels of 'healthy' HDL-cholesterol.[32–40] And anyway, the effect a diet has on cholesterol levels – or any other biochemical marker for that matter – is relatively irrelevant: it's the impact that a diet has on *health* that is really important. With regard to this, a recently published study found that women eating diets of the lowest GL were *half* as likely to suffer from heart disease compared to those eating high-GL fare.[41]

Other commonly expressed criticisms of low-carb diets relate to their high-protein nature, and the purported ability of protein to increase the risk of osteoporosis, kidney and liver disease. As we shall see in Chapter 8 (Lean Times), high-protein diets do not appear to have detrimental effects on bone health. Also, there is simply no evidence that supports the notion that high-protein intakes harm the liver or kidneys of healthy individuals.[42]

Another common concern about the restriction of starchy carbohydrates such as bread and breakfast cereals is that, in doing so, we will be missing out on much-needed nutrients. However, while it's often taken for granted that grains, particularly wholegrains like wholemeal bread, are packed full of nutrients, does this notion stack up in reality?

How Nutritious Are Grains, Anyway?

The nutritional value of foods can be measured in a number of different ways. One way would be simply to measure the levels of key vitamins and minerals in a food. While it makes sense for us to eat foods that offer a lot in terms of nutrients, some scientists believe that it can help at the same time if these foods are relatively low in calories. This has led researchers to develop a concept known as the 'nutrient density score'. Those foods with the highest nutrient density scores are those that are most likely to be truly nourishing to the body, without at the same time loading the body with excess calories.

In a study published in the *American Journal of Clinical Nutrition* the energy density and nutrient density score of some commonly eaten foods was assessed.[43] The nutrient density was based on the levels of 14 key nutrients (vitamins A, C, B_1, B_2, B_{12}, D, E, folate, calcium, iron, zinc, potassium and monounsaturated fat). Ideally, foods should have low energy density combined with high nutrient content. Let's have a look at the results for fruits and vegetables, and compare them to those of grain-based foods.

Figure 4.1 summarizes the results for fruits and vegetables. The healthiest foods will generally be those that are positioned low and to the right on the graphs. Looking at this figure, we can see that fresh fruits and vegetables, with the exception of the potato, rate very well indeed.

Now compare these results to those obtained for grains as seen in Figure 4.2.

As you can see, generally speaking grain foods are higher in energy density and lower in their nutritional offering. This graph has not specifically labelled refined carbohydrates such as regular pasta, white bread and white rice. However, you can see that, compared to fruits and vegetables, wholemeal bread turns out not very nutritious at all. In all likelihood, refined grains are going to be significantly worse. The bottom line is that while such fare can be described as food, it is actually better described as *fodder*.

It's also worth bearing in mind that some grains, notably whole wheat, contain substances called 'phytates' that actually block the absorption of nutrients such as calcium, magnesium, iron and zinc. So, not only do many grains lack much in the way of nutrients, they can actually *stop* us getting maximum nutritional value from other foods we eat them with.

Where Will I Get My Fibre From?

Another lingering concern regarding the reduction of starchy carbs in the diet relates to the fibre they contain. Wholegrains, such as bran-based breakfast cereals, wholemeal bread and brown rice are also relatively rich in what is known as 'insoluble' fibre or 'roughage', which we are told is essential for us to be able to open our bowels properly and help prevent colon cancer. In reality, as long as individuals are eating plenty of fruits and/or vegetables, there is usually no need at all for grains to be included in the diet

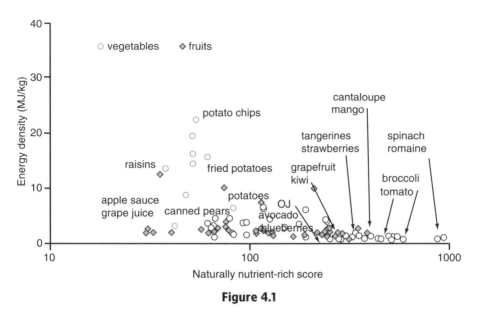

Figure 4.1

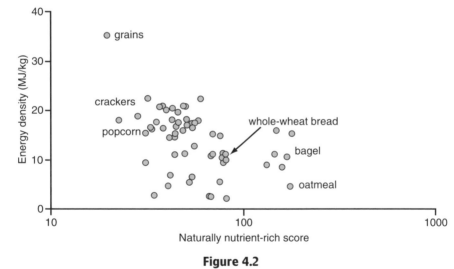

Figure 4.2

for healthy bowel function. And besides, studies have not proven that insoluble fibre has the capacity to reduce the risk of tumours in the colon.[44–6]

Food Fight

So grains, even in their unrefined form, turn out not to be the nutritional heavyweights they are so often made out to be. Bearing in mind this, and their generally disruptive effects on the body's chemistry, it doesn't look as though there's much in them to recommend. The news about grains gets even more unpalatable when we consider that some of them are a common cause of unwanted reactions to food, often referred to as 'food sensitivity' or 'food intolerance'. The mechanisms behind food intolerance are discussed in Appendix A. These reactions are a frequent factor in ill-health, and have often been found to be at the root of many cases of a wide variety of illnesses and conditions including irritable bowel syndrome, inflammatory bowel disease (such as Crohn's disease), fatigue, fluid retention, excessive catarrh and asthma.

While any food can, in theory, trigger such unwanted reactions, experience and some scientific evidence shows that some grains, particularly wheat, turn out to be common culprits. A likely reason for this relates to the fact that grains are a relatively recent addition to the human diet; this means many of us are not likely to be that well equipped to process them. Also, grains may contain substances (e.g. phytates) that inhibit the enzymes responsible for their digestion. This can only enhance the chance that these foods will go on to cause problems with food intolerance.

Of all the grains, wheat seems to be the worst offender of all. One reason why relates to the fact that the more we eat of a food, and the earlier it is introduced into our diet, the more likely we are to become sensitive to it. The fact is, many of us have eaten shed-loads of wheat in our lives, sometimes several times a day.

Not only that, but wheat is one grain that has been modified over the years using plant-breeding techniques. In other words, the type of wheat we eat now is often quite different from the wheat we originally started eating all those years ago. In short, it is likely that our bodies are simply less well adapted to the modern strains of wheat that pervade the modern-day diet.

Food on the Brain

The effect of partially-digested food seems to have the ability to extend beyond the body and into the brain. Once in the system, incompletely digested particles of food have the capacity to breech the brain's defences, where they may influence brain function and behaviour. The molecules concerned have what is known as an opioid-like effect, which means they influence the brain in a way reminiscent of opiate drugs such as morphine. One of the food components that can give rise to these so-called 'opioid-type peptides' is gluten (found most plentifully in wheat but also present in other grains such as oats, rye and barley).

One condition in which these reactions appear to be a potential factor is autism.[47] What is more, some evidence exists that suggests that excluding the foods most likely to give rise to increased levels of opioid-type molecules in the body and brain may actually reduce autistic symptoms.[48] My experience in practice has shown me that eating foods containing gluten can sometimes affect a person's general mental processes and mood. Lower mood and lack of focus and clarity are some of the more common symptoms that individuals suffering from this particular form of food reaction can experience.

So Why the Appetite for Grain?

The idea that grain-based foods have limited health benefits and can, in fact, pose significant hazards to our health seems to be in stark contrast to the enthusiasm health professionals and official bodies seem so often to have for these foods. To understand this disparity, we need to consider that grain is big business. There's a lot of money to be made in the growing of grain, and the food industry gets to spin this foodstuff into a dizzying array of cheap-to-produce and highly profitable foods such as bread, breakfast cereals, cereal bars, crackers, biscuits, pasta and savoury snacks. Notice that it is these very foods that have been developed into high-profile and instantly recognizable 'brands' including bread and breakfast cereals.

Part of the role of the grain and food industries, it seems, has been to convince health professionals and the unsuspecting public that these not-very-nutritious and potentially health-disruptive foods are healthier for us than nutritious, natural, unprocessed foods such as meat, fish, fruits, vegetables and nuts. Not only are these foods harder to brand, but they are simply not as profitable as the processed, grain-based fodder we are told should form the basis of our diet.

Should We Eat Grains at All?

I think the role of grains in the diet has been seriously overstated, but that does not necessarily mean we should not eat any of them at all. In the last chapter we looked at how there is evidence of adaptation to the consumption of dairy in some individuals who can digest the milk sugar lactose. The same, of course, could be true for grain.

My experience is that an individual's capacity to tolerate grain is tied into their biochemical individuality. In the Introduction to this book I introduced the concept of three broad types of people: the 'hunter' (who does well on animal foods rich in protein and fat); the 'gatherer' (who does well on a lower-fat, plant-based diet), and the 'hunter-gatherer' who is somewhere in between. We shall be learning more about these types of individuals, and what represents their ideal diet, in Chapters 12 (One Man's Meat), 13 (A World of Difference) and 15 (What Is There to Eat?). In general terms, the 'gatherers' tend to be best suited to grain, followed by the 'hunter-gatherers', and finally the 'hunters'. In Chapter 14 (Take the Test) you'll have the opportunity to discover your type and the place grain has in your diet.

However, because of their generally unnutritious nature and their ability to upset the chemistry of both body and brain, I do not recommend that anyone swallow standard dietetic advice and *base* their diet on grains.

I also think it's important to bear in mind that not all grains are created equal. If we are going to eat them, my suggestion would be to stick mainly to those grains that have relatively low GI, are unrefined, and are not particularly likely to provoke food-sensitivity reactions. With all these things in mind, I see oats, brown rice and whole rye bread as some of the healthier grains to consume.

Oats

Oats are reasonably slow sugar releasing, and generally come in a relatively unrefined form (e.g. rolled oats). Oats contain gluten, which is a common trigger of food intolerance. However, compared to other gluten-containing foods (e.g. wheat), oats seem in practice to be much better tolerated. Because they contain gluten, individuals with Coeliac disease (gluten sensitivity in the gut) are usually advised to exclude oats from the diet. Yet, evidence exists which suggests that certain Coeliac individuals can tolerate oats, despite the fact that they contain gluten.[49,50] This research supports the notion that oats are generally well-tolerated.

Brown Rice

Like oats, rice tends to be very well tolerated, and generally unlikely to trigger food-sensitivity reactions.

Whole Rye Bread

Whole rye breads generally have lower GIs and GLs compared to wheat-based breads. They also tend to be better tolerated from a food-sensitivity perspective.

Now that we've put grains in their place, we can go on to examine other recent additions to the diet. Next up is refined sugar and its supposedly 'healthy' counterparts: artificial sweeteners.

The Bottom Line

- Foods which give a substantial release of sugar into the bloodstream generally cause the body to over-secrete the hormone insulin.

- In the short term, surges of insulin can cause blood-sugar levels to drop, which may provoke symptoms such as fatigue in the mid-late afternoon, waking in the night and cravings for sweet foods.

- In the long term, excesses of insulin can promote weight gain and increase the risk of conditions such as heart disease and Type 2 diabetes.

- The extent to which a food destabilizes blood-sugar levels can be measured and is expressed as its 'glycaemic index' (GI).

- The overall effect of a food on blood-sugar and insulin levels will depend not just on its GI, but on how much of that food is eaten. This overall effect is described as a food's 'glycaemic load' (GL).

- Many grain-based foods including wheat bread, white rice, rice cakes and many breakfast cereals tend to have high GIs and GLs.

- Grains tend to be relatively low in nutritional value, even in their whole form.

- Some wholegrains, including wheat, contain substances that impair the absorption of nutrients such as calcium, magnesium, iron and zinc.

- Certain grains, particularly wheat, can cause problems with what is known as 'food intolerance'.

- Certain grains may also give rise to molecules called 'opioid-type peptides' that can impair brain function.

- 'Gatherers' tend to tolerate grains the best, followed by 'hunter-gatherers' and then 'hunters'.

- Some of the healthier grains include oats, brown rice, and whole rye bread.

Chapter 5 **Sweet and Sour**

Refined sugar is famed for its ability to rot our teeth, but evolutionary theory would suggest that this very new addition to the diet might have similarly corrosive effects deeper within the body. Our ancestors may have consumed some concentrated sugar in the form of honey from time to time. But what started as an occasional treat seems to have turned into a major habit: now a full 13 per cent of the calories we consume come from refined sugar in the form of foods such as soft drinks, confectionery, sugared breakfast cereals, sweetened yoghurts, desserts, biscuits and cakes.

One problem with refined sugar is that, apart from the carbohydrate it contains, it offers virtually nothing else from a nutritional perspective. Eating a diet rich in sugar could therefore cause us to miss out on nutrients that are key to our health and well-being. And in addition, as we discovered in the last chapter, sugary foods can have quite high glycaemic indices (GIs) and glycaemic loads (GLs), and may therefore have effects in the body that are none too sweet.

Sugar and Weight

The high-GI and -GL nature of sugary, processed foods mean that their consumption will tend to lead to surges of insulin. As we learned in the last chapter, this can stimulate the body to manufacture fat, and at the same time stalls the body's fat-burning abilities. In theory, then, sugar might possibly be helping to fuel the rise in rates of obesity.

The impact of sugar on weight was tested in one study in which individuals were asked to eat one of four diets.[1] One of these was high in fat. The other three diets contained much more in the way of carbohydrate. One of these was low GI, one was high GI, and the final diet was relatively rich in sugar (sucrose). Weight was found to fall on the low-GI diet, but increased on the other three diets. Importantly, though, the weight increase brought on by the high-sugar diet was nearly double that of the high-fat diet.

This is not the only research that has linked the consumption of sugar with increase in body weight. In one study, the relationship between the consumption of sugary soft drinks and weight was assessed in children. For each serving of soft drink, there was a whopping 60 per cent increased risk of obesity.[2] This evidence suggests, therefore, that diets rich in added sugar can indeed promote weight gain.

Sugar and General Health

Excesses of refined sugar in the diet may pose a hazard for our weight, but that's not the only hazard associated with this foodstuff. Other health issues related to sugar consumption include:

- the capacity to suppress immune function and reduce resistance to infection[3–5]

- the capacity to deplete the body of nutrients such as chromium and copper, while reducing the absorption of calcium and magnesium[6–9]

- the capacity to reduce the effectiveness of insulin in the body, thereby increasing the risk of raised insulin levels and Type 2 diabetes[10]

Can Excessive Sugar Consumption Lead to Type 2 Diabetes?

Eating and drinking sugary foodstuffs will generally cause considerable increases in blood sugar levels, which in turn can cause the pancreas to secrete excessive quantities of the hormone insulin (see Chapter 4 for more details about blood sugar and insulin balance in the body). In time, excessive insulin secretion can cause the pancreas to become 'exhausted', which may eventually lead to inadequate insulin levels in the body. Also, raised levels of insulin may cause the body to become less responsive to the effects of this hormone – a condition known as 'insulin resistance'. Inadequate insulin and/or insulin resistance may ultimately lead to the development of Type 2 diabetes. These mechanisms mean that, in theory, excessive sugar intake may increase the risk of Type 2 diabetes. In one study, the link between sugar consumption in the form of soft drinks and Type 2 diabetes was assessed in a group of 91,000 women followed over an eight-year period[11]. This research found that women consuming one or more can of sugary soft drink per day, compared to those drinking less than one can per month, were *twice* as likely to develop Type 2 diabetes.

Why Do the Official Recommendations on Sugar Consumption Lack Bite?

For a food that appears to have some considerable capacity to harm, recommendations for refined sugar's intake to be limited in the diet are surprisingly thin on the ground. For instance, in the official dietary recommendations of the US Institute of Medicine, published in 2002, it's advised that added sugars should not contribute more than 25 per cent of total calories[12] – that's about twice what we're currently eating.

Another example of the relatively relaxed attitude to sugar in the scientific establishment came in the form of a report prepared jointly by the United Nation's Food and Agriculture Organization (FAO) and the World Health Organization (WHO).[13] This report failed to confirm a link between the intake of sugars and chronic disease, and has been widely quoted as evidence that there is no established link between sugar and chronic (long-term) disease.

Bearing in mind its unhealthy properties, the official stance on sugar does appear quite permissive. And it seems this might well have something to do with politics and money. It has come to light that the FAO/WHO report cited above was secretly funded by the sugar industry.[14] Before the report was published the scientists who contributed to it met in Rome to discuss key questions, such as whether sugar is harmful to health. This consultation process was partly funded by two bodies known as the World Sugar Research Organization and the International Life Sciences Institute (ILSI) – both of which are funded by the sugar industry. It turns out that members of ILSI (an American research group funded by the likes of Coca Cola and Tate and Lyle) was able to recommend members of the committee and select the chairman, as well as review the agenda of the consultation.

One of the experts who took part in the preparation of the report, Professor Jim Mann from the Department of Human Nutrition at the University of Otago in New Zealand, is on record as exposing a worrying incident which occurred prior to the start of the consultation process. He described this episode in a documentary made by the BBC entitled *The Trouble with Sugar* which aired in 2004. A transcript of the documentary in which Professor Mann makes these revelations is available on line.[15] Professor Mann recounts during the documentary how he and some of his colleagues were summoned by one of the officials involved in organizing the consultation process, and were told that it would be inappropriate for them to say anything critical about sugar in relation to human health.

Bearing in mind these facts, I suppose it comes as no surprise that the FAO/WHO report was subsequently used by the sugar lobby to fight any suggestion of a link between sugar and ill-health. This rather sorry tale is an example of how the food industry has the capacity to pervert the course of science and to corrupt at the highest level.

Is Fructose the Healthy Alternative to Sucrose?

One type of sugar that is becoming increasingly prevalent in our food supply is fructose. This particular type of sugar is generally regarded as a healthier form of sugar when compared to sucrose (table sugar), essentially on account of the fact that it is said not to cause blood-sugar or insulin levels to rise. Also, fructose is to be found in fruit – something that tends to give a healthier image than sucrose, which is extracted from sugar beet or sugar cane.

Fructose has traditionally been seen in a favourable light as an added sweetener, and has generally been recommended as the sugar of choice for people with diabetes. However, studies show that fructose can impair the body's ability to handle sugar, and can reduce the effectiveness of insulin.[16] What is more, animal experiments reveal that long-term consumption of fructose can indeed lead to elevated levels of both sugar and insulin in the blood. These effects strongly suggest that fructose in the diet may predispose us to weight gain and diabetes.

One of the main food sources of fructose is fruit. Most fruits release their sugar relatively slowly into the bloodstream, which limits their capacity to disrupt the body's biochemistry and impair health. However, once fruit is juiced, the sugar becomes more available and therefore destabilizing. The sugar concentration of fruit juices is the same as soft drinks. And just like soft drinks, fruit juice can be glugged down in considerable quantities quite quickly. This can only add insult to the injury of fruit juice's highly sugary nature.

Fructose also finds its way into our diet as a food additive. For instance, soft drinks are often sweetened with high-fructose corn syrup. However, the evidence suggests that fructose as a food ingredient is likely to have effects as corrosive on health as sucrose, in the long term. This is likely to be particularly true for those who have difficulty handling sugar in the system. This is important, as fructose is often used as a sweetening agent in speciality foods designed specifically for people with diabetes.

While fructose generally enjoys a healthy reputation, there is good evidence it has the potential to harm our health. By all means include some fruit in your diet, but I would generally advise that fruit juices and foods with added fructose be treated with considerable caution.

Are Artificial Sweeteners All Sweetness and Lite?

Many people have cottoned on to the fact that refined sugar is not a substance to be consumed in quantity, and have moved more towards foods that have been artificially sweetened instead. These compounds are sweet but are virtually devoid of calories – what could be better?

There are several artificial sweeteners permitted in our food supply, including aspartame, sucralose, acesulfame potassium (also known as acesulfame K) and saccharin. The fact that these compounds are 'artificial', and are therefore *very* recent additions to the diet, should give us at least some cause for concern. On the other hand, the food industry is quick to repel any notion that artificial sweeteners are anything but perfectly safe, and to provide the science that supports this notion. For example, makers of aspartame (the most consumed sweetener in the UK diet) tell us that this compound is the most thoroughly tested substance in the human diet.

They'll also point to the 200-plus studies that prove that aspartame is fit for human consumption. A close look at the research, however, reveals that the scientific evidence is not as straightforward as some would have us believe.

Aspartame is composed of two amino acids (phenylalanine and aspartic acid), as well as a chemical entity that is known as a 'methyl' group. Once in the digestive tract, the body can digest aspartame down to its two amino acids, and the methyl groups end up being converted into something called 'methanol'.

All the major components of aspartame have been linked with adverse effects on health. Methanol, for instance, is a known nerve toxin. Within the body, it can be converted into formaldehyde – used for preserving dead bodies.[17] It has been demonstrated in animals that even low-level ingestion of aspartame can lead to formaldehyde accumulation in various parts of the body, including the liver and brain.[18] In addition, several human studies have found that chronic, low-level formaldehyde exposure has been linked with a variety of health issues including headaches and fatigue,[19–21] chest tightness,[22] nausea and lack of concentration,[23] seizures and behavioural impairment.[24] Aspartame consumption in humans has been found to induce physiological changes that might increase the risk of seizure.[25] In addition, at least one study has linked aspartame use with depression in individuals susceptible to mood disorder.[26] Other studies have linked aspartame ingestion with headaches.[27, 28]

So, while the food industry will give us supposedly soothing reassurances about the safety of aspartame, it seems that there's a fair body of evidence that runs contrary to this. What also concerns me is that whether a study finds in favour of aspartame or concludes that it does have potential to harm seems to be intimately related to one factor: who paid for the study. Evidence for this can be found in the form of an on-line review of aspartame safety studies.[29] Of 166 studies in this review, 74 had at least partial industry-related funding and 92 were independently funded. While 100 per cent of industry-funded studies conclude aspartame is safe, more than 90 per cent of independently funded research and reports show that aspartame has potentially toxic effects.

One reason for this disparity may relate to something known as 'publication bias'. Basically, the industry may choose to publish the results only of studies it likes the look of. Another explanation relates to the fact that many industry-funded studies seem to have been designed in a way that would make it unlikely for any harmful effects of aspartame to be detected. For instance, industry-funded studies have often given aspartame in the short term, many of them for a single day only. These methods in no way replicate the long-term, 'drip-feed' type of consumption many people experience in real life.

While long-term studies of the effects of aspartame have not been done in humans, these have been done in animals. In a recent study, Italian researchers fed aspartame in a variety of doses to rats over the long term.[30] The rats were given aspartame in their food supply from the age of eight weeks until they died. Rats consuming aspartame were found to be at significantly increased risk of several forms of cancer including lymphoma and leukaemia (cancer of the white blood cells). An increased risk of these conditions was found even at levels of aspartame intake lower than the official upper limit for humans. While in Europe intakes of 40mg of aspartame per kilogram of body weight per day are considered safe, an increased risk in cancer was seen in rats consuming just half this amount. My belief is that there is more than enough evidence to warrant exclusion of aspartame from the diet on safety grounds.

Does Aspartame Actually Help Weight Loss?

Even if you have your suspicions about the safety of aspartame, you might still resolve to consume it anyway, on the basis that this has to be better than sugar for your weight. After all, the promise with artificial sweeteners has always been that their very low-calorie nature is obviously less fat-promoting than something sugary. Bearing in mind aspartame's image in this respect, you might expect there to be a whole stack of scientific evidence attesting to this agent's effectiveness as a weight-loss aid.

Actually, the evidence for the supposed weight-related benefits of aspartame is conspicuous by its absence. To know definitively if aspartame is useful for those seeking to lose weight, it would need to be subjected to what is known as a 'double-blind placebo-controlled' study. In such research, individuals are randomly assigned to consume the substance being tested (e.g. aspartame) or something else (e.g. sugar). Neither the individuals in the study nor the investigators are allowed to know which individuals are having what. After some time, the 'code' is broken, the scientists find out who was taking what, and the results of the two groups are compared.

Curiously, to date, not one single double-blind placebo-controlled study designed to assess the effects of aspartame on weight has been published.

And there is even some evidence that aspartame ingestion may actually lead to *increased* food intake.[31,32] All this leaves me wondering why there is such enthusiasm from some quarters of the scientific establishment for aspartame as a weight-loss aid. The fact is, the evidence that aspartame is actually beneficial for weight loss is very thin on the ground.

If you're keen to get aspartame out of your diet, you may well steer clear of food products labelled 'diet', 'low-calorie', 'lite' or 'low-sugar'. However, you might need to do some serious label-watching, as aspartame is cropping up in more and more processed foods that do not advertise their low-calorie nature or suitability for slimmers. The reason? I don't know for sure, but it might have something to do with the fact that, for a given level of sweetness, aspartame is far cheaper than sugar.

Are Other Artificial Sweeteners Any Better?

One of the reasons I've focused on aspartame in this chapter is because it is the most studied artificial sweetener of all time. Aspartame has been the focus of literally hundreds of studies, and we can examine them to see just how poorly conducted much of the 'science' is, and how skewed a version of reality it seems the industry gives us regarding the safety and benefit of this artificial ingredient. Tellingly, aspartame has not been subjected to studies in which its long-term effect in humans has been assessed. Until such studies have been done, it seems premature to conclude that it is safe, especially when one considers the considerable body of evidence that points to aspartame's ability to cause harm. This absence of appropriate testing is true for all artificial sweeteners.

Of course, this would not be so much of an issue if they were not alien to nature. The fact that these substances are chemically synthesized and very recent additions to the diet means that it's highly unlikely that we have the appropriate biochemical or physiological machinery necessary to deal with them. What this means is that the chances that these agents will do us any good are small, and at the same time it means they may have considerable potential for harm.

Concerns about aspartame have caused food manufacturers to look for an alternative, and have found this in the form of the newer artificial sweetener known as sucralose. This substance is made by combining sugar with chlorine. The resulting compound is part of a chemical group known as the 'chlorocarbons', which includes the pesticides lindane and DDT.

Despite the strident reassurances regarding safety that come from the industry and the trade organizations, my advice is to avoid artificial sweeteners in whatever form they come.

The Bottom Line

• Refined sugar in the diet has been linked with a range of health issues including dental decay and an increased risk of weight gain.

• Recommendations regarding restricting sugar in the diet tend to be relaxed, though this may be because of political and commercial interference.

• Artificial sweeteners have not been sufficiently tested to be regarded as safe, and there is a considerable body of evidence that they have the capacity to have toxic effects in the body.

• There are no properly conducted studies which support the use of artificial sweeteners as an aid to weight loss.

• Overall, the evidence suggests that the consumption of both refined sugar and artificial sweeteners should be avoided.

Chapter 6 Slaying the Sacred Cow

Along with grains, dairy products such as milk, cheese and yoghurt represent a major staple in our diet. Many of us were introduced to dairy products very early on in life in the form of formula feed. And even if we were breast-fed, there's a good chance milk made its way into our diet quite soon after weaning. After all, our parents will almost certainly have had impressed on them the importance of milk and other dairy products as a source of much-needed calcium for the making of healthy bones and teeth. And females of all ages, of course, continue to be recommended to consume dairy products, lest they fall prey to osteoporosis in later life.

Yet, while the benefits of dairy products and their supposedly 'essential' role in the diet are often quoted, the relatively recent addition of these foods into the human diet should perhaps cause us to question the need for them in our diet. In the first chapter (What on Earth Did We Eat?) we learned that eating dairy products dates back just a few thousand years – a relative blink of an eye from an evolutionary perspective. And only very recently have we been 'processing' milk products through pasteurization.

Could these factors make giving dairy products a significant place in our diet a poor choice? We'll take a look at that notion later. Before that, let's start by asking what the rationale for eating dairy foods is, anyway. While we're repeatedly told that dairy foods are important for building healthy bones, is that really the case? Does this idea even make sense when one considers that, for practically all of our time on this planet, we made do without any dairy products other than our mother's milk?

Dairy – What Is it Good for?

Those keen to tout the benefits of milk will often highlight the fact that it is a prime source of calcium for building healthy bones. Particular emphasis, in this respect, is placed on the 'need' for children to consume foods such as milk and cheese. Because calcium is a component of bone and is found in dairy products, the theory is that these foods are important for making strong bones. But what *evidence* is there for this theory?

The role that calcium and dairy products play in bone-building was reviewed most recently in the journal *Pediatrics*.[1] In it, American researchers cast a critical eye over 37 relevant studies, of which 27 found no relationship between dietary calcium or dairy product intake and measures of bone health. Of the remaining studies, any apparent benefit was small. This review clearly deflates the notion that dairy products are 'necessary' for the normal growth and development of children.

Further evidence for the limited role of dairy products in building bone has come from a study published in the *British Medical Journal* which amassed evidence from 19 studies in the effects of calcium supplementation in children ranging from 3 to 18 years of age.[2] This mass of evidence found that calcium supplementation had no effect on bone density in the hip or spine, and very marginal benefits for bone density in the arm.

This study was accompanied by an editorial which highlighted the lack of evidence for the 'benefits' of not only calcium, but also dairy products generally, for bone health.[3] The editorial called for policy makers to revise calcium recommendations for young people and for a change in our assumptions about the role of calcium, milk and other dairy products in the bone health of children and adolescents.

The idea that drinking milk is not important for bone health in the younger generation may seem surprising to some, but this finding is very much in keeping with what we would expect from evolutionary theory.

Do Dairy Products Help Prevent Osteoporosis?

If dairy products don't do much for the bones of the young, have they anything to offer older folk? Dairy consumption has been widely advocated as the key component of a nutritional strategy designed to combat the bone-thinning disease known as osteoporosis. The role that milk, and the calcium it contains, have on bone health was assessed in a large study published in the *American Journal of Clinical Nutrition*.[4] In this piece of research, researchers tracked the dietary habits of 72,000 women for 18 years. Crucially, they found no relationship between the amount of milk and calcium a woman consumes and her risk of fracture of the hip. Put another way, drinking milk does not seem to strengthen women's bones.

In addition, a previous review of the literature found that 12 of 14 studies examining the relationship between milk consumption and bone health in women after the age of 50 found no association at all.[5] The concept that dairy products are important for ensuring healthy bones is one sacred cow worth putting to rest.

A Healthier Way to Healthy Bones

While the benefits of calcium, including that derived from dairy products, may have been overstated, having some of this nutrient in the diet is important for bone and general health. Good alternative sources of calcium include green leafy vegetables such as kale and broccoli. Veggies also tend to alkalinize the blood, something which appears to help preserve the calcium content of bone. Other good sources of calcium include tinned salmon and sardines. These are also rich in vitamin D – a nutrient that has an important role in the formation of bone. Another lifestyle factor where bones are concerned is exercise. Evidence suggests that weight-bearing activity has a much greater influence on measures of bone health than calcium intake.

Dairy Products and Food Sensitivity

In Chapter 4 (Against the Grain) we introduced a phenomenon known as 'food intolerance' and touched on how this may be at the root of a range of health issues including irritable bowel syndrome, asthma and eczema. In that chapter I pointed out that some grains, particularly wheat, are some of the most common offenders with regard to this problem. This phenomenon might be explained, at least in part, by the fact that grain foods are relative newcomers to the diet, and therefore are foods we are unlikely to be very well adapted to. Can you see where I'm going with this? Following the same logic, we should perhaps be suspicious of dairy products, too.

Experience in practice shows that dairy foods are a frequent factor in food sensitivity issues. I find dairy products are a very common cause in children of ailments such as asthma, eczema, ear infections, glue ear, frequent colds and recurrent tonsillitis. In adults, some of the most common symptoms include excessive catarrh, sinus and/or nasal congestion, asthma, eczema and irritable bowel syndrome.

One commonly recognized problem with dairy products relates to the sugar (lactose) they can contain. The inability to digest this sugar, called 'lactose intolerance', was explored in Chapter 3 (All Change). However, it's important to distinguish lactose intolerance with the types of reaction most commonly at the root of problems listed above such as asthma, eczema and sinus or nasal congestion.

The most common provoking factor here seems to be milk proteins such as casein. The theory here is that we are simply not well adapted to these proteins, don't digest them well, and can therefore leak them through the gut wall into the bloodstream, where they can trigger unwanted reactions. Critical to this issue seems to be the process of pasteurization. My experience in practice is that many individuals can tolerate raw dairy products, but react to those that have been pasteurized. Part of the explanation for this may lie in the fact that pasteurization can change the protein molecules in dairy products in a way that makes them harder to digest, and will therefore make them more likely to trigger unwanted reactions within the body.

Why Yoghurt Is Usually a Healthier Option than Milk

Interestingly, it is often found in practice that yoghurt is better tolerated than milk. Studies show that the bacteria used in the fermentation process that converts milk into yoghurt aid the digestion of milk proteins.[6,7] The pre-digestion of protein by these bacteria, and this helps to explain why, compared to milk, yoghurt is less likely to provoke food sensitivity reactions.

An added benefit of yoghurt is that some strains of bacteria used in making it have lactose-digesting ability, and thus yoghurt contains less lactose than milk. As a result, those who struggle to digest lactose generally find they tolerate yoghurt better than milk.

In addition to helping the digestibility of dairy products, studies suggest that the organisms found in 'live' and 'bio' yoghurts have the potential to help alleviate gut-related issues such as constipation, diarrhoea and irritable bowel syndrome. These beneficial bugs also seem to help keep the gut free from unwanted organisms including those responsible for food poisoning and the bacterium 'Helicobacter pylori' (the bug now recognized as a potential causative factor in digestive conditions such as stomach and duodenal ulcers, stomach inflammation and stomach cancer).

There is growing recognition that loss of healthy gut bacteria and an overgrowth of potentially unhealthy organisms, such as yeast or parasites, can cause symptoms within and beyond the gut. This problem, which is often referred to as 'gut dysbiosis', is covered in depth in Appendix B.

While I am a relative fan of yoghurt as a food, I advise avoiding 'fruit' yoghurts which, ironically, usually contain precious little fruit, and tend to be full of sugar and/or artificial sweeteners. My preference is for natural yoghurt, though there's no reason why this cannot be made more tasty and interesting – not to mention nutritious – with fresh or dried fruits, nuts, seeds and perhaps a spoonful of honey.

What about Other Dairy Products?

In practice, foods such as cheese and ice cream seem to have roughly the same potential as milk to induce food-sensitivity reactions. Butter, on the other hand, is generally very well tolerated indeed. This may have something to do with the fact that it is exceedingly low in the protein and lactose elements usually at the root of food-sensitivity reactions. The health effects of butter's main constituent – saturated fat – will be dealt with in depth in Chapter 8 (Lean Times).

Another common finding is that individuals who react to cow's milk-based products do not react as badly, or may not react at all, to products made from dairy products from other animals such as goats and sheep. Why this may be is not known for sure. However, it has been suggested that milk from these animals is, compared to cow's milk, more similar to human milk, thereby making it easier to digest and more appropriate for our consumption. Also, there is a school of thought which says that the earlier a food is introduced into the diet, and the more of it that is eaten, the more likely we are to become sensitive to it. While cow's products usually are consumed in quantity from early on in life, this is generally much less true for goat and sheep products.

I've seen many individuals shift from cow's products to goat's or sheep's products and do much better for it. More information about how to diagnose and manage food intolerance can be found in Appendix A.

Dairy Products and Opioid-Type Peptides

Another problem area we explored in Chapter 4 (Against the Grain) was the capacity for food to morph into molecules that can have a drug-like effect on the brain. One condition in which these compounds, often referred to as 'opioid-type peptides', have been implicated is autism. Opioid-type peptides come not only from grain foods containing the protein gluten, but also dairy products containing the protein casein. In Chapter 4 I made the point that opioid-type peptides seem to have the capacity to disrupt mental function in adults, too.

Curiously, it is well recognized in natural medicine that individuals often gravitate to the very foods that are having undesirable effects in the body. Could it be that the opioid peptides in gluten and casein are responsible for this? One thing that supports this theory is the fact that wheat and dairy products are quite often 'craved' by individuals sensitive to them. Some individuals, for instance, don't just *like* bread, but cannot imagine life without it. Others may feel they can't do without their cappuccinos or lattes, or have an unhealthy appetite for cheese. There is some indirect evidence that supports this concept in the form of research which shows that a desire to overeat appears to emanate from the same part of the brain that controls cravings in drug addicts.[8]

The Bottom Line

- Consuming milk and dairy products appears to have very limited benefit with regard to bone health in children or adults.

- Dairy products are a frequent cause of food intolerance-related conditions including asthma, eczema, and irritable bowel syndrome.

- Dairy products can have a drug-like effect on the brain, and this phenomenon may be a factor in conditions such as autism and food craving.

- Generally speaking, yoghurt and butter are better tolerated than milk and cheese.

- Goat and sheep dairy products are usually better tolerated than those based on cows' milk.

Chapter 7 **Oil Crisis**

In Chapter 3 (All Change) we explored the fundamental ways in which our modern-day diet differs from the typical hunter-gatherer fare that sustained us for some 2½ million years. In addition to grains, sugar and dairy products, we are now eating far more in the way of vegetable oils that have been extracted from foods such as sunflower seeds, rapeseed, corn and soya beans. Also, these fats can end up being processed in a way that gives rise to chemical entities which had no place in the diet until a few short decades ago. In this chapter we shall be taking a look at the nature of these fats, and seeing if their addition to our diet may help to explain the rise in the rates of chronic disease in recent times.

A Matter of Fat

Fat in the diet comes in several different biochemical types including 'saturated', 'monounsaturated', 'polyunsaturated' and 'partially hydrogenated' forms. Different types of fat have different effects in the body. Before we dissect these dietary constituents in terms of their health effects, we must first get clear on the terminology we shall be using when referring to these fats, and how this relates to their chemical characteristics.

The fats and oils in our food are composed of what are known as 'fatty acids' which are, simply put, made up of chains of carbon atoms with hydrogen atoms attached to them. The main classes of fat have subtle but important differences that distinguish them and their effects on health. What follows is a brief guide to the main fat types found in the diet.

Saturated Fats

The terms 'saturated', 'polyunsaturated' and 'monounsaturated' refer to the amount of hydrogen a particular fat contains. 'Saturated' fats, as their name suggests, contain as much hydrogen as they possibly can. These types of fats are found in animal products such as meat, eggs, butter, cheese, milk and cream, as well as in some non-animal foods such as coconut, palm and palm kernel oils.

Monounsaturated Fats

When a fat does not contain a full complement of fat, it is described as being 'unsaturated'. Hydrogen atoms go 'missing' from fats in pairs. When a fat is missing just two atoms of hydrogen it is called 'monounsaturated' fat. Foods rich in monounsaturated fat include olive oil, avocados and nuts and seeds.

Polyunsaturated Fats

Polyunsaturated fats have 4, 6 or 8 (or any other multiple of two) atoms of hydrogen missing. Polyunsaturated fats come in two main forms: the so-called 'omega-3' and 'omega-6' fats.

The main omega-6 fatty acid in the modern-day diet is known as 'linoleic acid'. Rich sources of linoleic acid include plant oils such as hemp, pumpkin, sunflower, safflower, sesame, corn, walnut and soya oil. Omega-6 fat also comes in the form of what is known as 'arachidonic acid' (AA), which is found in foods such as meat, fish and seafood.

The major omega-3 fatty acids in the diet come in the form of 'alpha-linolenic acid' (from plant sources such as flaxseed) as well as fats known as 'eicosapentaenoic acid' (EPA) and 'docosahexaenoic acid' (DHA), found mainly in oily varieties of fish.

Partially Hydrogenated Fats

These fats start out life as polyunsaturated fats and, as their name suggests, are then chemically processed to add some hydrogen.

The production of partially hydrogenated fats can result in the formation of related fats known as 'trans fatty acids' or 'trans fats'. The word 'trans' refers to the chemical shape of these molecules. In general terms, these fats are a different shape to fats found naturally, which usually come in what is known as 'cis' formation (see page 61).

Partially hydrogenated and trans fats can often be found in processed foods such as chips (French fries), fast food (such as burgers and chicken nuggets), margarine, biscuits, cakes, pastries and crackers.

In this chapter we're going to be focusing on the two fats that we are eating far more of nowadays than in the past – namely omega-6 and partially hydrogenated fats.

Omega-6 Fats

Just to recap, omega-6 fats are polyunsaturated fats that come in two main forms in the diet: linoleic acid (found mainly in plant oils such as hemp, pumpkin, sunflower, safflower, sesame, corn, walnut and soya oil and the foods from which these oils are derived) and AA (which is found in foods such as meat, fish and seafood).

As we discovered in Chapter 1, one of arachidonic acid's chief roles seems to be to 'feed' the brain. AA actually makes up more than half of the total amount of polyunsaturated fats in this organ. AA is believed to be important for visual function, too.

Omega-6 fats, both arachidonic and linoleic acid, are believed to have a wide range of functions in the body, which include effects on the health of the immune and cardiovascular systems. The biological effects of these fats is largely as a result of their conversion into hormone-like substances known as 'eicosanoids' (pronounced 'eye-coz-ah-noids'), which themselves come in a variety of forms (including substances known as prostaglandins, prostacyclins, leukotrienes and thromboxanes). These diverse chemicals can have a variety of effects on biochemical and physiological processes in the body.

Eicosanoids that come from the omega-6 fats tend to encourage physiological processes such as inflammation, blood-vessel constriction and blood-clotting in the body. As we shall see later, an excess of the eicosanoids derived from omega-6 fats are believed to increase the risk of conditions such as heart disease, stroke and arthritis.

Within the body, eicosanoids from omega-6 fats are balanced by the effect of those from omega-3 fats (e.g. the fats found in oily fish). The eicosanoids derived from omega-3 fats, generally speaking, tend to be anti-inflammatory in nature, and they have blood vessel-relaxing and blood-thinning effects, too. Because omega-6 and omega-3 fats have broadly opposing actions within the body, a 'balance' between these fats is vital for optimal health.

Our ancient diet did indeed contain foods rich in omega-6 fat such as meat, fish and nuts. However, only relatively recently did we start to consume much higher quantities of this fat in the form of cooking oils and fast and processed foods. Also, in our primal past we generally ate more in the way of omega-3 fats. It is estimated that the primal diet contained a ratio of omega-6 to omega-3 fats of about 1–3:1.[1] However, the fact that we are generally eating far more in the way of omega-6 fats and, almost certainly, less omega-3 too, has led to this ratio increasing to between 10:1 and 30:1 in a typical Western diet.[2]

What Is the Relevance of a High Omega-6:Omega-3 Ratio?

A glut of omega-6 fat in the modern-day diet may have important implications for our health. The higher the ratio of omega-6 to omega-3, for instance, the higher the risk of cardiovascular conditions such as heart disease and stroke.[3] Other evidence points to a raised omega-6:omega-3 ratio as a potentially important underlying factor in Type 2 diabetes.[4] This fatty imbalance has also been implicated in inflammatory conditions and autoimmune disease – conditions where the body's immune system reacts against its own tissues, such as rheumatoid arthritis.[5]

A major source of omega-6 fats are refined vegetable oils, which make their way into our food supply in foods such as fast food, margarine, biscuits, cakes, pizza, pastries, pretzels and corn chips. The evidence suggests that the dramatic increase we have seen in our intake of omega-6 fats is a potent force in the rise of many common health issues now seen in industrialized countries.

Eating fewer of these foods will probably have benefits for health, as will eating more omega-3 fats to balance their effect. The benefits of omega-3 fats are discussed in more depth in Chapter 9 (Animal and Vegetable).

Partially Hydrogenated and Trans Fats

The increasing amount of omega-6 fats in the diet is not the only change we have experienced in our fatty intake in recent times. Another shift has been in our intake of so-called partially hydrogenated fats. These fats are unknown in nature, and have only made their way into our mouths since the processing of vegetable oils got underway in a big way very recently. The hydrogenation of fats allows vegetable oils (such as sunflower and safflower oil) to be solidified, which is obviously critical in the manufacturing of solid fats such as margarine. The other 'benefit' of hydrogenation is that it makes fats less liable to turn rancid (go off), which extends their shelf life. The process of hydrogenation is good news for the food industry, but is it good news for *us*?

Again, evolutionary theory would suggest that foods containing partially hydrogenated fats would not make particularly good choices from a health perspective. In the last decade or so, scientists have focused their attention on the health effects of a particular type of partially hydrogenated fats known as 'trans fatty acids' or 'trans fats'. These fats are not only partially hydrogenated, but have also undergone an unnatural change in their molecular shape.

The polyunsaturated fats which are the raw material for industrially produced partially hydrogenated and trans fats are 'kinked' and even coiled in shape. The physical form of these fats is referred to as a 'cis' (pronounced 'siss') configuration. However, the processing of these fats not only adds hydrogen, but can also cause 'cis' fats to straighten out, forming what is known as the 'trans' configuration.

As expected, the research suggests that industrially produced trans fats have the potential for wide-ranging undesirable effects on health.

Trans Fats and the Heart

Trans fats have been linked with having adverse effects on heart health. For instance, in one study individuals who had suffered a heart attack were found to have significantly higher levels of trans fats in their bodies compared to healthy individuals.[6] Those with the highest concentrations of trans fat were found to be, on average, more than 2½ times more likely to suffer from a heart attack than those with the lowest levels.

A number of other studies also support the concept that trans fats are bad for the heart. Of four studies that have examined this potential association over time, three found that consuming just 2 per cent of our calories from trans fats is associated with an increased risk of heart disease of 28–93 per cent.[7–9]

Trans Fats and Cancer

Trans fats have also been associated with an increased risk of cancer. For instance, one piece of research found that higher levels of trans fats in the body were associated with an enhanced risk of cancers of the breast and colon.[10]

Trans Fats and Diabetes

Trans fats seem to have the ability to impair the function of the hormone insulin, something that would be expected to increase the risk of developing Type 2 diabetes.[11,12] Other research has found that, in women, a higher intake of trans fats is associated with an increased risk of diabetes.[13]

Trans Fats and Weight

There has not been much work that has examined the effect of the consumption of trans fats on body weight in humans. However, in one study, the effect of trans fats on weight was assessed in monkeys.[14] Here, one group of monkeys was fed a diet that contained 8 per cent of calories from trans fats. In another group of monkeys, the trans fats were replaced with monounsaturated fat. All monkeys in the study were fed the same total number of calories each day for a period of six years. At the end of the study, monkeys fed trans fats gained more than 7 per cent in body weight, compared to less than 2 per cent in the monkeys fed monounsaturated fat. Also, the trans fat-fed monkeys tended to accumulate their weight in and around the abdomen – precisely the form of weight gain most strongly linked with conditions such as heart disease and diabetes.

Trans Fat and Pregnancy

Trans fats also seem to have an association with adverse effects on pregnancy. One study, for instance, found that trans fats were associated with an increased risk of a condition called pre-eclampsia, which can lead to fitting in the mother.[15] Another study has found that higher levels of trans fats are associated with shorter pregnancies and lower birth weight.[16]

All in all, the evidence suggests – as we would expect from primal theory – that industrially produced trans fats are thoroughly unhealthy.

In the UK we consume an average of about 2.5–3.0 grams of trans fats per person each day.[17] This may not sound like much, except that studies show even very small amounts of these fats are associated with an increased risk of disease. In 2002, the Food and Nutrition Board of the Institute of Medicine in the US published a report on the role of trans fats on health, and made recommendations regarding safe levels of intake.[18] In the summary of this report, its authors suggest a 'tolerable upper intake level of zero'. In normal language, this translates as 'the safest amount of trans fats to consume is none at all.'

What about Trans Fats Found Naturally in the Diet?

Some natural foods, for instance butter, contain trans fats. The food industry sometimes refers to this fact, I suspect in an attempt to suggest that the industrially produced trans fats are somehow 'natural' too. However, industrially produced trans fats and those found naturally in food have different chemical constituents: industrially produced trans fats are predominantly monounsaturated trans fats, of which something known as 'elaidic acid' is a major component. Trans fats found naturally in food, on the other hand, are mainly in the form of very different fats known as 'trans vaccenic acid' and 'conjugated linoleic acids'.

Most importantly, studies suggest that it is the consumption of industrially-produced partially hydrogenated vegetable fat, rather than trans fat found naturally in food, that is associated with adverse health effects such as increased risk of heart disease.[19,20]

Is It on the Label?

Currently, in the UK there is no obligation for food manufacturers to declare the amount of trans fats their foods contain. However, they are required to list the partially hydrogenated fats from which they are derived during processing. Therefore, if you want to avoid trans fats, avoid eating any foods which have 'partially hydrogenated fat', 'partially hydrogenated oil', or 'partially hydrogenated vegetable oil' listed in the ingredients.

The Bottom Line

- The main fats found naturally in the human diet come in saturated, polyunsaturated and monounsaturated forms.

- Other, industrially produced fats in the diet include 'partially hydrogenated' and 'trans' fats.

- The polyunsaturated fats come in two main forms: omega-6 and omega-3. These have broadly opposing actions in the body.

- Our diet now has an omega-6:omega-3 ratio that is a lot higher than it was in our evolutionary diet, and this seems to increase our risk of a range of conditions including heart disease and arthritis.

- For better health, it makes sense to cut back on our consumption of omega-6 fats found in foods such as fast food, margarine, biscuits, cakes, pizza, pastries, pretzels and corn chips.

- Industrially produced trans fats seem to have a particularly detrimental effect on health, and have been linked with varied conditions including heart disease, diabetes, cancer and weight gain.

Chapter 8 **Lean Times**

While dietary advice can vary over time, one consistent message we've had from health professionals over the last few decades is the importance of cutting back on fat. The fat on which most attention has been focused is so-called 'saturated' fat – a constituent of foods such as red meat, dairy products and eggs. We are commonly warned that eating too much of this form of fat is almost guaranteed to cause the accumulation of fat in our body including within our arteries. Eating saturated fat, we are assured, is one sure way to pile on the pounds and increase our propensity to disability or even death as a result of heart attack or stroke.

One basic premise of *The True You Diet* is that a truly healthy diet will be, broadly speaking, one made up of foods that have been long-time components of our evolutionary intake. We have seen in the preceding chapters how foods that are relative newcomers to the diet, such as grains and dairy products, have a limited role in preserving our health. And very recent dietary additions, such as refined sugar, artificial sweeteners and trans fats, appear to pose significant hazards to those who consume them regularly.

Nevertheless, if the primal theory that underpins the dietary advice in this book is to hold true, then it doesn't make sense for saturated fat to be the toxic foodstuff it's cracked up to be. After all, saturated fat is a major constituent of meat – which in Chapter 1 we learned is a primal food if ever there was one. Either saturated fat is not the dietary spectre it's so often made out to be, or the primal theory on which this book is based is just plain wrong. Which is it?

To answer this question we're going to need to review the theories and examine the evidence for saturated fat's supposed unhealthy impact on the body.

Let's start with the commonly held belief that eating fat is a sure-fire way to get to *be* fat.

Does Eating Fat *Really* Cause Us to Be Fat?

One reason fat has a fattening reputation is because it is, well, *fat*. The idea here is that the fat we eat needs little chemical transformation before it is dumped as fat under our skin and elsewhere in our body.

Fat is also incriminated in the spiralling rates of obesity seen in so many countries because, weight for weight, it contains about twice as many calories as carbohydrate or protein. So, in theory, eating a lot of fat generally means consuming a lot of calories – something which one might expect to increase our risk of piling on the pounds.

While the theory that fat is fattening makes sense, if you've read the earlier portions of this book you'll know how much of conventional nutritional 'wisdom' turns out to be wide of the mark. So we may well ask: is the notion that eating fat causes us to *be* fat really how it is, or could it be a big fat lie?

Are All Calories Created Equal?

The concept that fat's calorific nature is inherently fattening is founded in the principle that eating more calories than we burn metabolically in the body will lead to weight gain. This 'calorie principle' forms the basis of pretty much all advice ever given to people wishing to lose weight. This usually translates into a blanket recommendation to those wanting to shed pounds: Eat less, exercise more.

When weighing up calorie balance in the body, most health professionals do not distinguish between different *types* of calories. In other words, the general view appears to be that a calorie is a calorie is a calorie, and that the form it comes in is quite irrelevant.

This obsession with calorie-counting seems to have blinded most of us to the fact that different types of calories are 'burned' differently in the body, and some burn more efficiently than others. We can think of the body's metabolism as rather like a fire which, say, easily burns small bits of dry wood, but has more difficulty with larger, soggy pieces of wood. Could it be that, for some individuals, eating fat is like putting small, dry pieces of wood on that fire?

One way to put this theory to the test is to assess the weight-loss effects of diets that contain the same number of calories, but are made up of varying amounts of fat, carbohydrate and protein. If it's really only the total number of calories that counts, then diets that contain the same number of calories should have the same effect on weight, irrespective of the composition of the diets. Actually, studies show this simply isn't the case.

In one study, for instance, the effects of two different diets were assessed in a group of women over a six-month period.[1] Each of these diets contained exactly the same number of calories, but one had 35 per cent of the calories coming from fat, compared to just 21 per cent in the other diet. In postmenopausal women, the women eating more fat lost significantly *more* weight (7.7kg versus 4.7kg).

In another study in women, the effects of a diet based almost entirely on carbohydrate was compared with one in which half the calories came from carbohydrate, with the other half coming from almonds (a fatty food).[2] Again, both these diets contained the same number of calories. Over 24 weeks, the almond-eating group actually lost 50 per cent more weight (an additional 7.2kg) than their carb-consuming counterparts.

In yet another study, this time in men, researchers compared three diets that contained the same number of calories but varied in the relative amounts of fat and carbohydrate they contained.[3] Individuals eating the most fat (and least carbohydrate) lost the most weight, while those eating the least fat (and most carbohydrate) lost the least.

What these studies show is:

- It's not just the number of calories we consume, but the form they come in that influences body weight.

- Eating a diet relatively rich in fat is not, in itself, a barrier to weight loss.

- Actually, all things being equal, eating more fat and less carbohydrate tends to lead to more effective weight loss.

This may seem utterly counter-intuitive when we bear in mind the fat phobia that many scientists and health professionals have engendered in us. However, remember that some individuals may, in theory at least, be quite efficient metabolizers of fat. In Chapter 12 (One Man's Meat) we shall dissect this theory in more depth and examine the scientific evidence for it.

Also, it is important to bear in mind that, through their effects on blood-sugar and insulin balance, certain carbohydrate foods have the capacity to promote weight gain. This was covered in depth in Chapter 4. Once we understand something about the effects foods have on our metabolism and physiology, we can see why it is that diets higher in fat and lower in carb than are traditionally advised can be effective for those seeking to attain or maintain a healthy weight.

More Reasons Why the Calorie Theory Falls Seriously Short

Apart from its failure to consider the *type* of calorie consumed, there is another reason why the calorie principle is seriously flawed. This concerns the effect foods have on appetite.

Some foods, while perhaps being low in calories, may do little to satisfy the appetite, and may therefore just lead to the consumption of more calories later on. On the other hand, a relatively calorific food may be highly effective in terms of quelling appetite, and may therefore lead to the consumption of less food later on. The ability of a food to satisfy our appetite clearly has important implications for weight and health in the long term.

As we learned in Chapter 4, the appetite-quelling effects of a food are influenced by the speed and extent to which it releases sugar into the bloodstream (known as the 'glycaemic index' or 'GI'). Basically, the lower a food's GI, the more satisfying it is. Foods rich in fat, such as meat and eggs, have very low GIs – something that will reflect well on their ability to sate our appetite. This is particularly the case for those of 'hunter' type (you'll be able to find out if this means you later in the book).

Another major component of high-fat foods such as meat and eggs is protein. Studies show that, calorie for calorie, this is the most appetite-suppressing component of the diet. This phenomenon is explored in more depth in the next chapter.

The notion that calorific foods, as long as they are low GI and protein-rich, can satisfy us in a way low-calorie foods may not be able to is not just theory, but has been shown in studies, too. In one piece of research scientists fed individuals 50g (320 calories) of almonds (a low-GI food rich in protein) each day for a period of six months to see what effect this had on weight.[4] During the almond-feeding period, the average weight gain was about 0.5kg – a small increase that was not statistically significant. Food diaries and interviews revealed that when individuals increased their consumption of nuts, they automatically compensated by eating less of other foods.

One final reason why the calorie principle doesn't stand up relates to the fact that the processing and metabolism of food within the body actually uses up some energy, and some foods use more than others. This, too, has implications for the propensity of a food to cause weight gain. As we learned in Chapter 4, this is particularly the case for protein. It is perhaps worth bearing in mind that many natural foods which may be high in fat, such as meat and eggs, are also rich in protein.

Just How Effective Are Low-fat Diets Anyway?

Never mind all this theory, though – the only way to know if dietary fat is a potent force in obesity is to test this with appropriately designed studies. One suitable type of study would be to put people on high-fat diets to see if they gained weight. As we've just seen, studies show that diets higher in fat seem to speed weight loss. Also, don't forget that in Chapter 4 we looked at a bunch of evidence which shows that low-carb diets (which are often also high in fat) can lead to satisfying weight loss.

The more conventional way of testing the impact of fat on weight, of course, is to assess the effectiveness of low-fat diets. What does the science show with regard to such studies?

Before we look at the results, it is important to consider that the best test of a low-fat diet would be to compare it with another diet which does not explicitly restrict fat (sometimes referred to as a 'control' diet). Generally, in these studies, individuals assigned to eat the low-fat diet are given more instruction and support than those in the 'control' group. This will generally give results that favour the low-fat diet. Now let's look at some studies that have assessed the effectiveness of low-fat eating.

In one study, fat intake was reduced from 38 to 20 per cent of the total number of calories in the diet of a group of women.[5] Two years later, the difference between those eating the lower-fat diet and those on a control diet was an average of 1.8kg. This is better than nothing, perhaps, but one might argue that this is a pretty paltry result for all the sacrifice and deprivation required to restrict fat quite dramatically in the diet.

Also, there is some evidence that when weight is lost on a low-fat diet, not all weight lost is composed of fat. This was shown in a study of overweight women on a reduced-fat intake. In this case, fat was limited to provide about 18 per cent of total calories.[6] This quite extreme restriction of fat led to an average weight loss of an additional 2.6kg compared to a control group. However, lean tissue (such as muscle) was lost as well as fat. A year into the study, the difference in change in body fat percentage between the two groups was less than 1 per cent.

Now remember, in these studies low-fat dieters are generally given more advice and support, which can bias results in their favour. To counter this effect, researchers in one study gave those assigned to the low-fat and control diets similar amount of instruction.[7] The result? No significant differ-ence between results achieved by the two groups.

The evidence from individual studies suggests that low-fat diets have little or no benefit over diets that are richer in fat. In order to get an idea of the overall effect of low-fat eating on weight, several relevant studies were assessed in a review published by the highly-respected international group of researchers known as the Cochrane Collaboration in 2002.[8] The researchers were particularly interested in the ability of participants to sustain weight loss over a long period of time.

The average amount of weight lost in low-fat and control diets was assessed at 6, 12 and 18 months. The Table below summarizes the findings of this review.

Table 8.1

	Average weight change on low-fat diet (kg)	Average weight change on control diet (kg)
6 months	– 5.08	– 6.50
12 months	– 2.30	– 3.40
18 months	+ 0.1	– 2.30

You can see that any initial weight loss seen on a low-fat diet declines in time. This was also true of the control diets, but not nearly to the same extent. In fact, the control diets out-performed the low-fat diets at every stage. And perhaps most importantly of all, at 18 months those instructed to eat low-fat diets had, on average, actually *gained* weight, while those eating control diets had lost some. This is not the only review of the evidence to find that low-fat diets are less effective than control diets where weight loss is concerned.[9] In the long term, it seems that all the sacrifice and deprivation usually entailed on a low-fat diet gets people precisely nowhere.

Whatever you may have been told, the science shows that cutting back on fat is simply ineffective for the purposes of weight loss in the long term.

Saturated Fat and Heart Disease

In addition to its influence on weight, saturated fat is often maligned for its ability to clog up our arteries and boost our chances of succumbing to conditions such as heart disease and stroke. While this notion is perhaps deeply embedded in our collective psyche, we will know by now how important it is to review the evidence for even the most deeply entrenched nutritional 'facts'. So, where did the idea that saturated fat causes heart disease come from, and is this concept as scientifically sound as it's so often assumed to be?

The notion that fat has any relationship at all with heart disease seems to have been born about half a century ago. In 1953, an American researcher by the name of Ancel Keys published a study which compared the fat consumption and risk of death due to heart disease in six countries.[10] This research showed that the more fat eaten in a country, the higher the risk of heart disease. Keys followed this study up with a much bigger study where the dietary habits and health of men in seven countries (Finland, Greece, Italy, Japan, Yugoslavia, the Netherlands and the US) were assessed over a 10-year period.[11] This study specifically analysed the relationship of not just fat, but *animal* fat, and heart disease. The results of this research showed that, generally speaking, the more animal fat eaten in a country, the greater the overall risk of heart disease.

Studies like these seem, on the face of it, to be pretty convincing evidence that eating saturated fat is a risk factor for heart disease. However, before we jump to any conclusions, it's important to bear in mind that Keys' studies are what are known as 'epidemiological' in nature. This type of research essentially analyses the relationship between factors (such as diet or exercise) and health. The problem is, even if an association between two things is found, this does not prove that one is *causing* the other. For example, studies have found that owning a car is associated with an increased risk of heart disease. It's unlikely, though, that owning a car actually *causes* heart disease. More likely it is other factors associated with car ownership, such as a tendency to be less physically active and perhaps increased weight, that are the true culprits. So, even though original studies may have shown an association between saturated fat and heart disease, they simply cannot be used to conclude that saturated fat actually *causes* heart disease.

It's important to remember this particularly because Keys' research compared individuals living in different countries. Lifestyle habits tend to vary a lot between countries, and it could be these differences (and not differences in fat intake) that might explain variation in heart disease risk. For this reason, more accurate judgements are gained by comparing individuals *within* a country. Tellingly, Keys' research found that death due to heart disease varied widely between regions within a country, despite similar dietary habits. This suggests that fat has much less influence on heart disease risk than is generally suggested.

Another major deficiency with Keys' original work was that it appears he was quite selective about the data he presented. When he originally published his 1953 study, there was information from not six countries around the world, but 22. When *all* the data available at the time is analysed, the association between fat intake and heart disease basically disappears. Could it be that Keys might have been deliberately selective about the data he used to prove his point? We'll never know for sure, but it sure looks that way.

What's Happened Since?

Despite these glaring deficiencies in Keys' work, the concept that feeding ourselves saturated fat is a major risk factor in heart disease was vigorously taken up by the scientific and medical establishments. And the concept is full of life today. You might therefore expect that there has been plenty of other evidence that supports Keys' original contention.

Over the last half-century or so there have been more than two dozen studies that have analysed the relationship between saturated fat and the risk of heart disease.[12–37]* All but four of these studies found no association between saturated fat intake and heart disease.[38] And in one study, higher intakes of saturated fat in the diet were found to be associated with *reduced* narrowing of the arteries supplying blood to the head (the carotid arteries) over time[39] – something that is taken as a sign of reduced risk of cardio-vascular disease.

---

*Information in this section has been adapted from Colpo A, *The Great Cholesterol Con* (Lulu.com, 2006)

The largest analysis to date of the relationship between lifestyle factors and risk of heart attack was published in the *Lancet* medical journal in 2004.[40] This study analysed a range of risk factors and heart attack risk in some 12,000 heart attack victims and 14,000 healthy individuals from 52 countries around the world. The researchers involved in this study identified several factors, including smoking, high blood pressure, diabetes, a low intake of fruits and vegetables, and low levels of physical activity that appeared to account for 90 and 94 per cent of heart attacks in men and women respectively. Curiously, this review makes no mention of animal fat, or even dietary fat in general, as being an important risk factor for heart attack.

Taken as a whole, the scientific evidence simply does not support the notion that saturated fat is bad for the heart. And don't forget, even the scant evidence that exists which supports a link is 'epidemiological' in nature, which means that it in no way could ever prove that saturated fat *causes* heart disease.

In order to ascertain whether saturated fat might actually cause heart disease, it is necessary to perform what are known as 'intervention' studies. This essentially means putting people on low-saturated fat diets to see what effect this has on their risk of heart disease.

Ideally, studies of this nature should be double-blind, which means that neither the individuals in the study nor the researchers will know whether they are receiving the true intervention or not These sorts of studies are generally regarded as the gold standard of intervention studies. To date, only two such studies have been performed with regard to heart disease risk or death,[41,42] and neither showed any benefit.

There are 20 other relevant studies,[43-62] of which just six[63] found benefit. So, of a total of 22 studies, 16 found no benefit for the heart from cutting back on saturated fat.

This doesn't seem like particularly convincing evidence of the supposed benefits of eating less saturated fat. And the evidence looks even less convincing when you consider that the studies that *did* find benefit are often what is known as 'multiple-intervention' studies – which in this case means that, in addition to reducing saturated fat, the participants were subjected to at least one other modification. For example, in one study individuals were given nutritional supplements.[64] In two of the studies, individuals were asked to emphasize heart-healthy omega-3 fats as well as fruit and vegetables in the diet.[65] The obvious question that multiple-intervention studies raise is whether lowered saturated fat in the diet, or the other interventions, or a combination of these things, is what proved effective. Because of these limitations, multiple-intervention studies cannot be used to judge the effects of reducing saturated fat in the diet.

One way researchers can get a good idea of the overall effect of some treatment or approach is to perform what is known as a 'meta-analysis'. Here, results from a number of similar studies are grouped together. The largest meta-analysis to examine the effect of modifying fat in the diet was conducted by UK-based researchers and was published in the *British Medical Journal*.[66] This particular review amassed the data of 27 individual studies. Neither deaths due to cardiovascular disease (such as heart attack and stroke) nor overall risk of death was found to be reduced by changes to intake of dietary fat.

The results of this review support the notion that eating less saturated fat has little, if any, benefits for our heart or general health.

So What's the Point of Eating Less Saturated Fat?

Eating less saturated fat is generally regarded as a key to good health. However, low-fat eating has been shown to be ineffective for the purposes of weight loss in the long term, nor does it protect us from disease. So, what really is the point of eating less saturated fat? It seems that the point is: there is no point!

It is, of course, possible to over-consume saturated fat. A diet, say, made of nothing but butter would not be a healthy one. Such a diet would lack the nutritional variety necessary for good health. By the same token, a diet based on broccoli would not be a healthy one either. The important thing here is that *saturated fat is not inherently unhealthy, and therefore does have a place in a healthy diet*.

As we shall see in Chapter 12 (One Man's Meat), some individuals have a greater capacity to cope with fat in the diet than others. 'Hunters' are best suited to this foodstuff, while 'gatherers' do least well on it. Later on you'll get the opportunity to find out what type you are, and from this you'll be able to judge the appropriateness of saturated fat in your own diet.

Saturated Fat and Cholesterol

The lack of evidence that saturated fat is bad for the body, and the evidence that it indeed may have benefits for health, has not necessarily dented the

Saturated Fat's 'Healthy' Primal Nature

We have examined the science and discovered that saturated fat has, if anything, a broadly benign effect on health. While this obviously runs counter to the anti-fat propaganda many of us will be familiar with, this is in keeping with the primal and evolutionary theory of healthy eating. Saturated fat, after all, is a constituent of meat – a food we have been eating for pretty much all of our time on this planet, and therefore something we should be quite well adapted to by now.

Then again, if saturated fat is such a long-time constituent of the diet, one might expect it to have positively *beneficial* effects on health. For a start, saturated fat is a critical component of a substance called 'phospholipid' which is the primary constituent of the walls of our cells. What this means is that saturated fat plays a crucial role in the structural integrity of all our cells. Looking at it like that, saturated fat suddenly seems to offer much more than the weight-boosting and artery-clogging effects it is infamous for.

Other evidence points to saturated fat as a positive health-giver. Some research, for instance, has suggested that saturated fat is the preferred form of fuel for the heart.[67] Other evidence suggests saturated fat may have a range of beneficial effects in the body including anti-cancer effects,[68,69] as well as antimicrobial action including an ability to combat bacterial and viral organisms.[70-73] Taking a broad view of the effects of saturated fat in the body, it seems it does have benefits for our health after all.

enthusiasm health professionals seem to have for advising us to cut as much of it as possible out of our diets. In recent years, advice to reduce saturated fat has often referred to its ability to raise the levels of cholesterol in the bloodstream. And this, we are told, can increase the risk of atherosclerosis – the artery-clogging process that increases our risk of conditions such as heart attacks and stroke.

There is indeed some evidence that high cholesterol levels are associated with an increased risk of heart disease and death, though a close look at the available evidence shows that this association only seems to be true for individuals up to the age of about 50 or so. After that time, plenty of evidence shows that 'raised' cholesterol levels in later life are not associated with adverse effects on health.[74-88] Indeed, there is even some evidence that higher cholesterol is actually associated with enhanced longevity and survival.[89-92]

Now, it's worth bearing in mind that the vast majority of cases of conditions said to be related to raised cholesterol levels (namely heart attacks and strokes) occur in middle age and beyond. As the science shows that cholesterol is not a risk factor, and indeed may even be beneficial, in people of this age, then this should perhaps cause us to question the current appetite to paint cholesterol as the culprit.

As with saturated fat, if we really want to make a judgement of the true impact cholesterol has on health, we need intervention studies – studies in which cholesterol levels are lowered and the effect of this assessed. In 2005 a meta-analysis of 17 studies in which subjects made dietary changes explicitly to reduce blood cholesterol levels was published in the *Archives of Internal Medicine*.[93] Overall, these studies brought about a 10 per cent lowering of cholesterol levels. Despite this, the amassed results showed no reduced risk of death, neither in healthy individuals nor even in high-risk individuals who had a history of heart attack or stroke. Basically, taking dietary steps to reduce cholesterol levels simply does not seem to save lives – yet more evidence that cholesterol is not as important a factor in health as it is so often said to be.

What about the Benefits of Cholesterol-reducing Drugs?

Apart from diet, the other major way to quell cholesterol levels is through drug therapy. Currently, the most popular type of medications used for this purpose are known as the 'statins' which include atorvastatin (Lipitor), rosuvastatin (Crestor) and simvastatin (Zocor). A huge stash of cash has been made out of these drugs, but is their life-saving reputation deserved?

Statins do seem to have the capacity to save lives, though the benefits seem to be largely confined to individuals who already have diagnosed cardiovascular disease (e.g. heart disease or previous stroke). This evidence is often used to support the notion that cholesterol causes heart disease. However, in addition to reducing cholesterol, statin drugs also have other effects in the body that would be expected to reduce the risk of cardiovascular disease. For instance, it is well recognized that statins have anti-inflammatory effects, and current evidence suggests that inflammation is an important underlying process in the development of cardiovascular disease. This has raised the question that statins' apparent ability to reduce the risk of cardiovascular disease may have nothing at all to do with cholesterol.

Now, that doesn't mean that these drugs should not be used. It does mean that we should be clearer about how they exert their effect, and whether cholesterol-reduction is truly beneficial.

And just how effective are statins, anyway? These drugs are often said to reduce the risk of heart attack by about a third. This may sound impressive, but the risk of heart attack for most individuals is actually very small. Why don't we give newborn babies statins? Because they are at zero risk of heart attack. However, a lot of adults can have very low risk of heart disease too, which means that reducing their risk by a third won't make much difference in real terms.

This is particularly important for individuals who have no history of cardiovascular diseases such as heart disease or stroke, and are therefore generally at low risk of these conditions. When essentially healthy individuals are treated with statins, this is called 'primary prevention'. Current recommendations mean that many individuals with 'raised' cholesterol levels may end up on a statin despite being fit and healthy, and perhaps without being at any real risk of cardiovascular disease. How much are statins likely to help these individuals?

A meta-analysis of seven trials in which statins had been used in primary prevention was published in the *Archives of Internal Medicine*.[94] It did find that the risk of heart attacks and strokes was reduced by 29 and 14 per cent respectively. However, statin therapy did not reduce the risk of death due to heart attack, nor the overall risk of death. What this study shows is that for essentially healthy people, statins do not appear to save lives.

One way to get a good idea of how effective a treatment really is in practice is to measure something known as the 'number needed to treat'. Such studies essentially ask questions like: 'how many individuals would need to be treated for five years to prevent one death due to heart disease?' This is precisely the question that was asked by researchers who were assessing the number needed to treat for national cholesterol-reducing programmes in several countries including New Zealand, the US, Canada, and the UK.[95] This study found that the number needed to treat ranged from 108 to 198. So, at their best, more than 100 people would have to be treated for five years with statins to prevent one death. At their worst, the number needed to treat is more like 200.

Now, for the one in 100 to 200 people who evades a fatal heart attack by taking statin medication, the drug has been, quite literally, a life saver.

However, let's also consider for a moment the 100 to 200-odd other people for whom statins have had much more limited benefit. Let us not forget that drugs have potential side-effects, too. Statins, specifically, are known to deplete the body of a naturally occurring nutrient known as coenzyme Q10. In time, this can lead to symptoms that include generalized fatigue, muscle weakness and pain. More serious reactions are also known to exist, though these are typically not reported in trial results. And we need to bear in mind the cost of these drugs, naturally.

Looking at this data might cause some to question why statin drugs have been embraced with such enthusiasm by the medical establishment.

My suspicion is that the answer has a lot to do with money. Statin drugs are a source of considerable revenue for the pharmaceutical industry. It seems that the heavy promotion of statin drugs, and selective quoting of data regarding their relatively limited benefits, has had an influence that extends far and wide.

One example of this concerns the decision to make the statin simvastatin available over the counter (OTC) in the UK in 2004. This decision seemed an odd one, bearing in mind that there is little, if any, evidence that statin therapy helps more than a small minority of the general population. Also there has simply been no analysis at all of the likely effects of simvastatin use as an OTC medication. The Government body instrumental in making this decision was the Medicines and Healthcare Products Regulatory Agency (MHRA). The MHRA had previously stated that in the consultation process that preceded the licensing of simvastatin as an OTC medication, about two-thirds of respondents were in favour of this practice. This turned out to be a gross distortion of the truth – the reality was that only about one third of individuals asked were in favour. The MHRA put this 'mistake' down to 'administrative error'.

The year 2004 also saw the introduction of recommendations to use increasing doses of statins to 'optimise' cholesterol levels. This directive came from a panel of nine scientists, eight of whom were subsequently revealed to have financial links with drugs companies making statins. The report's publisher described the omission of these clear conflicts of interest as an 'oversight'. I'll say.

I suppose this wouldn't matter too much if the recommendations to lower cholesterol limits were based on good science. The scientific basis of these recommendations was reviewed in a study published in the *Annals of Internal Medicine* in 2006. The authors of this review state: 'In this review, we found no high-quality clinical evidence to support current treatment goals for [LDL] cholesterol.' They went on to say that the recommended practice of adjusting statin dose to achieve recommended cholesterol levels was not scientifically proven to be beneficial or safe.[96]

Of course all this focus on cholesterol as a killer is not just good for the drug industry, but the food industry, too. Food manufacturers have been happy to clamber onto the cholesterol bandwagon by offering a plethora of foods that can be labelled as 'low in cholesterol', or 'cholesterol free', as though that somehow confers some health advantage. Of late, the food industry has also branched out into the provision of foods that are sold with the promise that they will help reduce our cholesterol levels.

Perhaps the most obvious example of this is the specialized margarines that contain plant compounds called 'stanols' or 'sterols'. These help block the absorption of cholesterol from the gut, and can therefore help to reduce cholesterol levels in the bloodstream. The very fact that taking dietary steps to reduce cholesterol has never been shown to save lives should cause us to doubt the supposed benefits of these specialized margarines. But what about margarine in general? Does this food really deserve to be branded as healthier than butter, as the manufacturers and marketers would have us believe?

Is Margarine *Really* Better than Butter?

For some decades now, margarine has been marketed as a 'healthy' alternative to butter. Initially, margarine was sold to us on the basis that, compared to butter, it was lower in saturated fat. This selling proposition obviously rests on the assumption that saturated fat is *bad* for health. Earlier in this chapter, though, we discovered that the science suggests this simply isn't true.

The other claim made for some types of margarine, as we have just discussed, is that they help reduce cholesterol levels. Even if cholesterol-reduction through dietary means had been proven to be beneficial (which it has not), would that mean something that reduces cholesterol is automatically healthy? I mean, if arsenic and cyanide were shown to have cholesterol-reducing properties, would it make sense for us to be consuming these substances every day? This may sound a bit extreme, but let's see what goes into making margarine.

The major constituents of this spread are 'vegetable' oils, obtained from foods such as sunflower seeds, rapeseed or soya beans. These oils are usually extracted using the application of pressure and heat, and maybe the use of solvents, too. This processing can damage the fats and impart some unhealthy properties on them. The oil obtained by this process is then treated with sodium hydroxide to 'neutralize' certain fats in the oil that are unstable and may cause spoilage. The oil is then bleached and has any 'impurities' removed by subjecting it to a substance known as fuller's earth (a clay-like material). The oil is then filtered to remove this bleaching and cleansing agent. After this, the oil is subjected to steam treatment to remove unwanted odours. The end result of this process is essentially colourless, flavourless, and liquid.

To convert this into margarine, more processing is obviously necessary. To make liquid oils solid they may be subjected to chemical processes such as 'inter-esterification' or hydrogenation. Inter-esterification involves the use of high temperature and pressure, along with enzymes or acids, to 'harden' the oil. In hydrogenation, hydrogen is bubbled through the oil at high temperature. Both processes have the potential to make fats that are quite unknown in nature – something that should give us considerable cause for concern with regard to their effects on our health. More information about partially hydrogenated fats can be found in Chapter 7.

And we're not done yet. After this, the solidified fat that we now have is generally blended with other fats, which can be of vegetable or animal origin. After this, the product needs to be both coloured and flavoured. Then, what are known as 'emulsifying agents' are added to prevent the product from separating out. And finally, the end product is extruded into a plastic tub for our delectation and delight. Is this sounding like a food you want to put in your mouth, never mind swallow?

Also, compare margarine's alien-to-nature nature to butter, which is basically made from the fat found in milk. Half of butter's weight comes from saturated fat, while about 20 per cent of it comes from monounsaturated fat, which is believed to have positive heart-healthy properties. Apart from the addition of some salt, butter is a relatively natural, unprocessed food, the main elements of which have likely been a constituent of the human diet since the very beginnings of our evolution. And it tastes better.

Once individuals know these facts about margarine and butter, my experience is that there are few who don't intuitively feel that butter is a better bet. However, so effective has the marketing and promotion been, it

> **What About Margarines Made from Olive Oil?**
>
> Olive oil is principally composed of monounsaturated fat, which is generally believed to have heart-healthy properties. However, once such fat has been subjected to the sort of chemical manipulation necessary to convert it into margarine, the chances that it will retain any healthy properties are remote to say the least. Plus, this type of margarine would also contain substances that may be positively detrimental to health. This particular form of margarine is likely to be as inappropriate for our consumption as any other.

can be hard to let go of the belief that margarine is healthier than butter. So, what evidence is there for this?

Well, we've already seen that the lower levels of saturated fat and ability to quell cholesterol levels do not seem to confer any benefits. And even if they did, the important thing to assess is not these factors, but the effects of margarine and butter on *health*.

To know for sure whether margarine really is healthier than butter, we would need to have the results from double-blind placebo-controlled trials (trials in which individuals are given butter or margarine to eat, though neither they nor the researchers are allowed to know which). After some time, the researchers would then assess which group, if any, had the better health outcome. Unfortunately, no such studies have been published.

There is, however, one study in the scientific literature which examined the association between butter and margarine consumption and risk of heart disease in men.[97] This study found that butter consumption was not associated with heart disease risk. In other words, those men eating more butter were not at increased risk of suffering from heart disease. On the other hand, margarine consumption *was* associated with heart disease – it appeared to *increase* risk: in the long term, for each teaspoon of margarine consumed each day, risk of heart disease was found to be up by 10 per cent. That means that, in the long term, eating 3–4 teaspoons of margarine a day is associated with a 30–40 per cent increased risk of heart disease.

So, if at any point you should come across a message or piece of advice that compels you to eat margarine rather than butter, my suggestion is: Don't swallow it.

The Bottom Line

- Saturated fat, a constituent of foods such as red meat and dairy products, has a reputation for causing weight gain and increasing our risk of heart disease.

- The idea that saturated fat causes weight gain is based on the fact that, weight for weight, fat contains about twice as many calories as either protein or carbohydrate.

- However, the *form* a calorie takes has a bearing on how efficiently it is 'burned' in the body.

- Studies show that when total calorie input is the same, diets higher in fat (and lower in carbohydrate) tend to promote more effective weight loss than diets low in fat (and higher in carbohydrate).

- Foods high in fat may also be high in protein – an element of the diet which tends to be effective for quelling appetite.

- Studies show that low-fat eating is ineffective for the purposes of weight loss in the long term.

- Although research dating back more than 50 years found a relationship between fat-eating and heart disease, the majority of studies do not support this association.

- Reducing saturated fat in the diet does not appear to have broad benefits for health.

- Saturated fat appears to have some benefits for health, including an anti-microbial effect and the ability to supply fuel for the heart.

- The evidence shows that saturated fat has a place in a healthy diet.

- While eating saturated fat can cause cholesterol levels to rise, in later life raised cholesterol levels do not seem to be associated with an increased risk of heart disease, and can even be associated with increased longevity.

- Taking dietary steps to reduce cholesterol has not been shown to save lives.

- Cholesterol-reduction through drug treatment is of limited benefit, particularly in those who are healthy.

- There is no evidence that margarine is healthier than butter. In fact, some evidence suggests that margarine is associated with an increased risk of heart disease, while butter is not.

- Margarine is a wholly unnatural, highly processed and chemicalized food, for which no evidence exists to support its 'healthy' reputation.

- Butter is an ostensibly natural food, the main constituents of which have been part of the human diet for ever.

Chapter 9 **Animal and Vegetable**

So far in this book we have charted the human diet over the course of our evolution, and discovered that relative nutritional newcomers such as grains, refined sugar, artificial sweeteners, dairy products and refined and processed 'vegetable' oils have little or no part to play in a truly healthy diet. On the other hand, we have discovered that saturated fat – a primal food if ever there was one – simply does not have the devastatingly toxic effects its reputation would suggest. If anything, this fat seems to have a number of benefits for human health.

In this chapter we're going to extend our examination to the major evolutionary foodstuffs that survive to this day in the modern-day diet: meat, fish and seafood, eggs, fruits, vegetables, nuts and seeds. We shall also take a look at beans and lentils, which, while not what you'd call 'primal' foods, nevertheless have some positive nutritional attributes that allow them some place in the diet, especially for 'gatherers'.

Once we have explored the nutritional attributes of each of these foods, we will then take a look at the evidence (or otherwise) for the widely held notion that vegetarian diets are inherently healthier than those that are more omnivorous in nature.

Meat

Meat, particularly red meat, has been branded as an unhealthy food for as long as most of us care to remember. This reputation has mainly been based on meat's content of saturated fat – a 'forbidden' foodstuff that science shows actually does have a place in a healthy diet.

Another component of meat that is often in the firing line is cholesterol. However, as we saw in the preceding chapter, the role of cholesterol in ill-health seems to have been seriously overstated. Also, bearing in mind that taking dietary steps to reduce cholesterol has not been shown to save lives means that there seems to be little point in losing sleep over this particular form of fat, either.

Saturated fat and cholesterol are not the only forms of fat to be found in meat – another is monounsaturated fat, found in foods like olive oil and avocado, generally taken to have heart-healthy properties. The monounsaturated fat content of meats like beef and lamb is not inconsiderable either: levels of monounsaturated fat in these foods are almost identical to levels of saturated fat.[1]

There's a bit more to meat than fat, of course. Actually, pound for pound, meat (including red meat) contains substantially more protein than fat. Dietary protein is composed of chains of molecules known as amino acids, which are the building-blocks used in the manufacture of many structures and tissues in the body including bone, muscle, skin, nails and hair. Protein is essential for normal growth and development in children, and in adults provides the raw materials necessary for body maintenance and repair.

Protein may also be of critical importance for those wanting to lose weight. How so? Well, calorie for calorie, protein has been found to satisfy the appetite more than either carbohydrate or fat, which may be critically important in weight control.[2] Also, as we saw in Chapter 4, the processing of protein in the body uses up a fair amount of energy for free.[3]

In one study, the effect of two diets that differed in protein content was studied with regard to their effects on appetite and weight.[4] Individuals participating in this study were first of all prescribed a calorie-controlled diet of which 15 per cent of calories were contributed by protein (with 35 per cent of calories coming from fat) for two weeks. After this, the diet was changed to one which contained the same total number of calories as the first diet, but which now had 30 per cent of its calories contributed by protein (and 20 per cent of calories coming from fat).

The researchers found that despite contributing the same total number of calories, the higher-protein diet led to significantly increased feelings of fullness and reduced hunger compared to the lower-protein diet. The subjects were then instructed to continue to eat this higher-protein diet for a further 12 weeks, but this time with no restriction placed on how much they could eat. During this phase individuals naturally ate less and ended up losing an average of 5kg.

Another of protein's benefits concerns its effects on the *type* of weight that is lost. This is relevant because when individuals lose weight, not all of it, unfortunately, will be fat. There is the potential for muscle to be lost, too, and this has important implications in the long term as our 'muscle mass' has considerable influence on our overall metabolism. As muscle is made primarily of protein, it stands to reason that eating a protein-rich diet might actually help to preserve muscle mass during weight loss. And that's exactly what a review of 87 relevant studies has found.[5]

It should perhaps also be borne in mind that, as we discovered in Chapter 3, the level of protein in the Western diet is significantly lower than that found in more primitive hunter-gatherer diets. This suggests that our needs for protein are actually significantly higher than we are currently consuming.

Protein and fat, along with carbohydrate, represent the three so-called 'macronutrients' in the diet. Macronutrients, as their name suggests, are required in the body in much greater quantities than other substances found in the diet known as 'micronutrients' which include vitamins and minerals. Now that we've dealt with the two major macronutrients in meat, let's turn our attention to those micronutrients.

What Else Is in Meat?

Perhaps the most famous micronutrient in meat is the mineral 'iron'. This nutrient is an essential component of the constituent of red blood cells called 'haemoglobin' that carries oxygen around the body. Iron deficiency can cause of low haemoglobin levels (anaemia), which can lead to a serious sapping of our sense of mental and physical well-being. What is less well recognized is that, irrespective of its role in making haemoglobin, iron participates in reactions which generate energy in the body. A low level of iron can, therefore, cause symptoms such as fatigue and low mood, even if it does not cause anaemia.

In my experience, iron deficiency is not uncommon, and people at risk of it include women (maybe as a result of iron loss in menstrual blood and some tendency to avoid red meat in the diet), vegetarians and vegans. The best test for iron levels in the body is the serum (blood) 'ferritin' level. However, the normal levels for ferritin are set very wide, which means that someone with 'normal' but low levels of iron can still suffer with symptoms of iron deficiency. In my experience, individuals will usually not experience optimal levels of energy until their ferritin level is above about 50 ng/ml.

Those seeking to enhance their iron levels have diet and supplements at their disposal. With regard to this, it may be useful to bear in mind the fact that the form of iron found in meat and other animal foods (known as 'haem' iron) is much more absorbable and useable by the body than the form of iron found in plant foods (known as 'non-haem' iron). Generally speaking, I do not find iron supplements particularly useful for raising ferritin levels, partly because the forms of iron found in them can be relatively difficult to absorb. One exception seems to be the liquid forms of iron found readily in health food stores. High levels of iron can be damaging to the body, so I do not advise iron supplementation unless testing has revealed low or low-normal ferritin levels. Monitoring of ferritin levels over time is also important to ensure that iron levels in the body do not rise too high.

Another mineral found in good quantity in meat is *zinc*. This nutrient plays an important role in, among other things, immune function, wound healing, brain function and fertility. As far as vitamins are concerned, meat offers a rich complement of B-vitamins, including B_1 (thiamin), B_2 (riboflavin), B_3 (niacin), B_6 and B_{12}. These nutrients have a wide range of functions in the body, and assist both in the generation of energy and in balanced brain function.

Another of meat's nutritional offerings comes in the form of *carnitine* – a substance comprised of the amino acids lysine and methionine. One of carnitine's chief roles is to help the conversion of fat into energy in the body's cells.

In stark contrast to its traditional image, meat's macronutrient and micronutrient profiles reveal it to be a nutritional heavyweight.

Meat Quality

Any reservations I have about meat are related not so much to the food itself, but to the methods used to rear the animals that give up their meat, and to any processing that may occur afterwards. Many commercially reared animals are intensively farmed, and often exposed to drugs and chemicals that taint their meat and may have undesirable effects when subsequently consumed by humans (especially children). One of the worst meats in this respect is chicken. While poultry is generally regarded as healthier than red meats such as beef and lamb, this is not necessarily the case. Most chickens are kept in miserable conditions and loaded with growth-promoting antibiotics during their brief lives. Some chicken-processors go on to add

Is Protein Really Bad for Our Bones?

Protein may have natural appetite-suppressing properties and be critical to body regeneration and repair, but not everyone is enthusiastic about its consumption. One major qualm about protein relates to its purported effect on bone. A diet rich in protein has the capacity to increase acidity in the bloodstream, in response to which the body will tend to liberate calcium from the bone. 'Evidence' for this comes from studies which show that when individuals eat protein, levels of calcium in the urine go up. Over extended periods of time, this supposed leaching effect of calcium from the bone is said to increase our risk of osteoporosis and fracture.

However, while it is often assumed that the calcium losses in the urine that follow eating protein come from its loss from our bones, some research has shown that protein in the diet increases the absorption of calcium from the *gut*. This mechanism provides an alternative explanation for why a high-protein diet can cause calcium levels to rise in the urine, and also opens up the possibility that protein may actually help supply the body with the calcium it needs for optimal bone formation. Also, protein itself is an important component of bone – something which often seems to get missed.

In a study published in the *American Journal of Clinical Nutrition* researchers examined the relationship between protein consumption and bone health in more than 1,000 women.[6] Higher protein intakes were associated with improvements in both the bone density in the hip and the quality of the bone in the heel. This study is actually part of a considerable body of research which has explored the relationship between protein intake and bone health. While the findings of these studies are not utterly consistent, most studies have found that higher protein intakes are associated with generally better bone density.

proteins from other animals (such as cows and pigs) to the meat to help its retention of added water. Chicken is one meat that is almost certainly worth eating in its organic, free-range form. The same is also true of pork, which is another usually intensively reared meat. Going organic is probably the best option for other meats such as lamb and beef, though I think this is generally less of a concern as these animals are usually less intensively reared. Other options include game meats such as venison, partridge, pheasant and duck.

Also, there is evidence that the type of feed an animal eats during its life has a bearing on the nutritional profile of the meat it gives up. Animals like cows and sheep are adapted, essentially, to eating grass. Yet in the intensive rearing of animals grass is often substituted with grain (which is not these animals' natural diet at all). Compared to grain-fed animals, those that have been grass fed end up having high levels of the omega-3 fats which have been associated with a range of benefits for body and brain.[7] More about these eminently healthy fats can be found later on in this chapter in the section on fish.

The processing of meat is another potential concern. There is a big difference between an unadulterated organic chicken breast and a chicken nugget. The latter is likely to contain poor-quality meat, a range of additives and maybe some particularly unhealthy trans fatty acids, too. Also, processed meats such as hot dogs may contain preservative chemicals such as sodium nitrite. In the stomach, sodium nitrite can combine with amino acids to form substances known as 'nitrosamines', which research shows have cancer-causing potential. For instance, a study published in the *Journal of the National Cancer Institute* found that approximately two of every five cases of stomach cancers appeared to be caused by sodium nitrite.[8] In other research, nitrites have been linked with an increased risk of brain tumours.[9]

Another form of cancer that is often said to be related to meat-eating, particularly red meat, is colon cancer. The evidence in this area, though, is inconsistent. For instance, a review of the available literature published in the *European Journal of Clinical Nutrition* found that of 44 relevant studies, most (31) found no apparent association between red meat intake and colon cancer risk.[10] This review suggested that any heightened risk of colon cancer comes mainly from eating processed meats (such as sausage and salami), as well as meat cooked at high temperatures (e.g. chargrilled and barbecued meat). Some more evidence for the proposed role of processed foods in colon cancer came from a study published in the *International Journal of Cancer* in 2002, which found that, pound for pound, processed meat has significantly more cancer-causing potential in the colon than red meat.[11]

In a more recent review, both red meat and processed meat consumption were associated with an increased risk of colon cancer.[12] One of the problems with this review, however, is that it did not take account of other factors related to colon cancer such as, say, vegetable consumption. If, for example, someone eating nothing but red meat were at increased risk of colon cancer compared to someone who also ate plenty of vegetables, the enhanced risk wouldn't be down to the red meat itself but to the absence of protective vegetables. Basically, this most recent review cannot be used to discern whether the apparent link between eating red meat and colon cancer is actually due to the red meat itself, or to other factors *associated with* eating red meat, such as, say, consuming fewer vegetables.

What I think is almost certainly true is that if we're going to eat meat, then it makes sense to choose cuts from animals that are as naturally reared as possible. And, as a general rule, I recommend that the bulk of any meat we eat should be in an unprocessed form. To my mind, hunks of meat like steak, lamb and organic chicken are, generally speaking, to be preferred to things like sausages, ham, bacon or salami.

Another step in the right direction with regard to meat is to buy it from a farm shop, farmers' market or local butcher where the origin of the animal is more likely to be assured. Using your purchasing power in these places also helps support the local economy.

And finally, while meat is broadly beneficial from a health perspective, not all individuals do equally well on it. As we shall see in Chapter 12 (One Man's Meat), red and fatty meats are particularly appropriate for 'hunter' types and, to a lesser degree, 'hunter-gatherers'. Less fatty forms of meat (such as chicken breast) tend to be more appropriate for the 'gatherers'.

Eggs

Eggs, along with red meat, have generally been caught up in the anti-fat hysteria that most of us will be familiar with. However, we now know that saturated fat and cholesterol are not to be feared. Besides, the most plentiful type of fat to be found in eggs is actually of the monounsaturated variety – a type of fat associated with a reduced risk of heart disease. Again, as with red meat, this fact is rarely mentioned when health professionals have a crack at eggs.

There are studies in the scientific literature which have linked egg-eating and heart disease. At the risk of sounding repetitive, such studies (termed 'epidemiological' studies) may show an association between two things, but that does not mean one *causes* the other. The association may be due to other factors (known as 'confounding' factors) that have not been taken into consideration. The reason for pointing this out again is that the studies linking egg-eating with an increased risk of heart disease have traditionally not accounted for possible confounding factors. When studies *have* taken them into consideration, however, the evidence suggests that intakes equivalent to an egg a day are not associated with an increased risk of heart disease in men and women free from diabetes.[13] This sort of threshold does seem to fit with primal theory. While it is highly likely that we foraged for eggs during our evolution, this food almost certainly did not contribute substantially to the diet.

Eggs are a good source of protein, and this may be particularly valuable for vegetarians. Eggs are also relatively rich in vitamin B_{12}, which is also potentially useful to vegetarians whose options for getting enough of this important nutrient are limited.

One potential concern regarding eggs is that they are quite a common cause of food-sensitivity reactions, often referred to as 'food intolerance'. In my experience, eggs are not nearly as likely to trigger reactions as other foods such as wheat and cow's milk, but their role in food intolerance is commonplace enough for it to warrant mention. More information about the diagnosis and management of food intolerance can be found in Appendix A.

Fish and Seafood

Fish and seafood (such as prawns, crab and mussels) are generally healthy foods that offer good-quality protein and may also supply the body with other beneficial nutrients. These foods are, for instance, a good source of zinc – some of the benefits of which were covered in the section on meat, above. Fish and seafood are also rich in iodine, which has a critical role to play in the health of the thyroid gland – an organ that has a vital role to play in well-being and general health. (For more about the role of the thyroid in health, see Appendix D.) One other common constituent of seafood and fish is vitamin D which, among other things, has an important part to play in bone and muscle health, as well as protecting the body against cancer and helping with mood regulation, too.

Any information about these and other nutrients to be found in fish and seafood tends, these days, to be swamped by the tide of information that comes at us regarding the so-called omega-3 fats contained in these foods.

In Chapter 7 we discovered that compared to our evolutionary diet we are eating far fewer omega-3 fats in comparison to so-called omega-6 fats, and discovered how this may be fuelling rates of chronic disease. In addition to cutting back on omega-6 fats, another obvious way to redress this imbalance is to consume more in the way of fats of the omega-3 variety.

Much of the press about omega-3 fats focuses on the benefits they have for the heart and circulation. These fats, found most abundantly in fish such as salmon, trout, mackerel, herring and sardines, have the capacity to thin the blood, reduce blood pressure and help maintain a normal heart rhythm – all things that would be expected to translate into reduced risk of heart attack, stroke and a condition known as 'sudden cardiac death'. One review of 50-odd studies concluded that omega-3 fats, either from oily fish or fish-oil supplements, have the capacity to reduce death rates due to heart disease, as well as overall risk of death.[14]

The benefits of omega-3 fats seem to extend beyond the body and into the brain, too. One of the two main types of omega-3 fats found in fish is called docosahexaenoic acid (DHA). DHA is believed to play an important part in the structure of the brain. Higher levels of this fat in the body have been linked with a reduced risk of dementia.[15] The other type of omega-3 fat found in fish is known as eicosapentaenoic acid (EPA). EPA seems to contribute to the day-to-day running of the brain. Higher levels of this fat are believed to help ward against a variety of ills including depression, dyslexia and hyperactivity. If you cast your mind back to the first chapter (What on Earth Did We Eat?), you may remember that some scientists believe that the eating of omega-3 fats (from foods such as fish, brain and bone marrow) appears to have been a critical factor in the development of a larger brain and the subsequent evolution of our species.

However, as with meat, some questions have been raised about potential contaminants to be found in fish. Mercury, for instance, is quite commonly found to taint fish such as tuna, marlin and swordfish, and has the potential to cause neurological damage. Fish, particularly farmed fish, may be contaminated with substances such as 'dioxins' and 'polychlorinated biphenyls' (PCBs) which are believed to have cancer-promoting effects in the body. Look deeply enough and no food is perfect, and this includes fish. This makes it important, wherever possible, to assess the overall effects of a food on health. When this was done, the conclusion was that eating fish does more good than harm.[16]

Another potential cause for concern where fish is concerned is the depleted fish stocks in our seas. As a result, fish-farming is now increasingly being used to meet demand (and generally at a lower price, too). Fish-farming generally involves exposing fish to chemicals (such as antibiotics and colourings) that are not encountered in the wild. Also, fish-farming is bad news from an ecological perspective.

In an ideal world, fish is best consumed in wild rather than farmed form. However, fresh fish is generally expensive, and we need to be mindful of the depleted fish stocks in our seas. For a guide to the best fish to eat from a sustainability and ecological perspective, see www.fishonline.org.

Canned fish, though not as good as fresh from a nutritional perspective, represents a more cost-effective way of consuming fish. The most popular canned fish in the UK is tuna. Tuna is often referred to as an 'oily' fish. However, while fresh tuna does contain some omega-3 (though not nearly as much as fish such as salmon and mackerel), much of this is removed before canning. Tuna is also one of the fish, along with marlin and swordfish, that tends to be contaminated with mercury (see above). Better types of fish to have from a can are salmon, mackerel and sardines. These are richer in omega-3 fatty acids, and tend not to be contaminated with mercury.

As we shall explore in Chapter 12 (One Man's Meat), 'hunter' types tend to do well on 'oily' varieties of fish such as salmon, sardines and mackerel, while 'gatherers' tend to do best on non-oily fish such as cod, haddock and plaice.

Now that we've weighed up the pros and cons of the major animal foods, we can turn our attention to the plant-based foods such as fruit, vegetables and nuts.

Fruit and Vegetables

Along with grains, fruits and veg tend to feature highly in recommendations for a 'healthy' diet. However, in contrast to grains, fruit and vegetables have generally lower glycaemic indices and loads – something that would be expected to give them a considerable nutritional edge over grains. The perils of consuming a diet rich in foods of lofty GI and/or GL were covered in depth in Chapter 4 (Against the Grain). Also in that chapter we saw how, compared to grains, fruits and vegetables pack much more of a nutritional punch.

Fruit and vegetables are well known for their ability to supply the body with health-giving nutrients such as vitamin C and folate. Plant foods such as these also offer the body a relative cornucopia of substances known as 'phytochemicals' (also known as 'phytonutrients') which have considerable disease-protective potential. Black grapes, for instance, contain the phytochemical resveratrol, which studies suggest may help protect against cancer and heart disease. Hesperidin, a phytochemical found in citrus fruits, is believed to stave off heart disease. Apples and onions are rich in substances called 'flavonols', which are linked with a reduced risk of heart disease, while strawberries and other berries offer a phytochemical by the name of 'ellagic acid' which research suggests has significant cancer-protective properties. What are known as 'cruciferous vegetables' (which include broccoli, cabbage, Brussels sprouts and cauliflower) have been found to contain sulphur-containing compounds that have the ability to assist in the detoxification of cancer-causing agents known as 'carcinogens'. This is just a small sampling of the literally hundreds of phytochemicals found naturally in fruit and veg.

Bearing in mind the range of nutrients that fruits and vegetables offer, it is perhaps no surprise that eating them is associated with a reduced risk of diseases such as heart disease and cancer. One major report concluded that diets high in fruits and vegetables (intakes of more than 400 grams per day) could prevent at least 20 per cent of all cancers.[17]

The Potato – A Vegetable in a Class of its Own

Vegetables are generally healthy for all types of people, but one exception is the potato. Unlike most other vegetables, the potato has a relatively high glycaemic index and load, which is not such a good thing, as we saw in Chapter 4 (Against the Grain). It is also a vegetable that tends to offer little in the way of nutritional value compared to other vegetables such as leafy greens. For these reasons, potatoes do need to be consumed with some care by all individuals, especially 'hunters'.

However, while potatoes are not an ideal vegetable, they do have at least some things going for them (in addition to their versatility, that is). Studies have found that, compared to foods such as bread, rice and pasta, boiled potatoes have much more capacity to satisfy the appetite.[18] And, from a food-sensitivity perspective, potatoes tend to be much better tolerated compared to certain grains, especially wheat.

As with lots of other foods, not all types do equally well on potatoes. In general terms, they suit 'gatherers' more than 'hunters'.

Other research has focused on the effect of fruit and vegetable consumption on cardiovascular diseases such as heart disease and stroke. In one study, consumers of fresh fruit were found to be at significantly reduced risk of heart disease, stroke and overall risk of death.[19] In other research, intake of vegetables has also been found to be associated with protection from heart disease.[20] Fruit and vegetables have been linked with a reduced risk of other conditions too, including osteoporosis[21] and eye conditions such as cataract and macular degeneration (the most common cause of blindness in the elderly).

Does it Pay to Go Organic?

Whilst fruits and vegetables should assume a generally prominent place in our diet, there is always the potential that they will come laced with unwanted chemicals. A lot of fresh produce is quite liberally treated with agrochemicals such as pesticides and fungicides that are designed to keep it free from attack by insects and moulds. How do we know these things are safe? We *don't*. The toxicity studies done in animals used to set safe levels in no way reproduce real life. Essentially, each one of us is engaged in an experiment in which we are consuming a cocktail of chemicals for years or even decades. This may be deemed appropriate by the authorities, but common sense dictates that the fewer of these chemicals we consume, the better.

With this in mind, I do regard organic fruit and vegetables as a healthier option than regular fare. Not only are they less likely to be contaminated with harmful chemicals, but there is some evidence that they may contain higher levels of nutrients including vitamin C and phytochemicals, too. The benefits of organic produce are comprehensively dealt with in a 2001 report commissioned by the Soil Association entitled *Organic Farming, Food Quality and Human Health* (see www.soilassociation.org).

While organic produce is the best choice for a number of reasons, its often premium price can put it beyond the reach of many. Very thorough washing of fresh produce will at least help to reduce the negative impact pesticide residues may have on health.

Nuts and Seeds

Nuts are an intensely fatty food, something that generally causes them to have an unhealthy reputation. While about 80 per cent of the calories nuts offer comes from fat, much of this can come in the so-called monounsaturated form believed to have benefits for the heart and circulation. Nuts are also rich in nutrients such as magnesium, potassium, copper and vitamin E – all of which may also have benefits for cardiovascular health.

Given their nutritious nature, it is perhaps no surprise that eating nuts has been associated with a reduced risk of heart disease. One study found that women consuming at least 5 ounces (about 125 grams) of nuts each week had one-third fewer heart attacks compared to women who rarely or never ate nuts.[22] In another study, men eating nuts twice a week, compared to those who rarely or never ate nuts, were found to be at about half the risk of a condition known as 'sudden cardiac death'.[23]

Seeds (e.g. pumpkin, sesame, sunflower) have not been formally studied with regard to their effects on health. However, because they are nutritionally very similar to nuts, we would expect them to have broadly similar benefits for the heart.

One of the main reasons some individuals avoid eating nuts is because they are very fatty, so the assumption is that they must be *fattening*. However, in the last chapter (Lean Times) we saw how eating fat is not necessarily fattening, and may even aid weight loss. Nuts, in theory at least, should burn reasonably efficiently in the body on account of their supremely primal nature. There is indeed evidence to support this, in the form of a study in which men were asked to eat 500 calories-worth of peanuts (peanuts are technically a legume – see Beans and Lentils on page 98 – but have a nutritional profile very similar to nuts) every day.[24] At the end of the 19-week long study, resting energy expenditure (basically, the metabolic 'idle speed' of the body) had risen by more than 10 per cent. This is proof that when we put the right sort of food into the body, it can actually stimulate the metabolism, just like putting some dry wood on a fire.

Also, being rich in protein we would expect that nuts may be effective in sating the appetite, which could just lead us to eat less of other foods. Many individuals find that eating some nuts in between meals, for instance, can help stop them overeating at meal time. So, what does the evidence show? In a review published in the *European Journal of Clinical Nutrition*, 13 individual studies looking at the effect of nuts on weight were assessed.[25] All the studies in which nuts were used to replace other foods found no increase in weight. However, what is perhaps more surprising is that even when nuts were added to an existing diet, all but one study found no tendency to lead to weight gain. Nuts may be fatty, but the evidence strongly suggests they are not *fattening*.

While nuts are broadly healthy, their fatty, protein-rich nature makes them more appropriate for 'hunters' and 'hunter-gatherers' than 'gatherers'.

Beans and Lentils

Beans and lentils are collectively referred to as 'pulses' or 'legumes'. The term 'legume' comes from the fact that these foods are seeds of plants belonging to the 'leguminosae' family, which have a pod that protects the seeds while they are forming and ripening.

There seems little doubt that beans and pulses were only introduced into the human diet relatively recently – probably about the same time as grains, about 10,000 years ago. Like a lot of grains, legumes seem to have some capacity to trigger food-sensitivity issues. One component of legumes that may be responsible for these unwanted reactions are food components called 'lectins'. Legumes also contain substances that impair the action of digestive enzymes in the gut such as amylase and trypsin.[26] These 'enzyme inhibitors' impair the digestion of food, which can increase the risk of food sensitivity and may reduce the nutritional value that can be derived from food, too.

There is some evidence that the lectins and enzyme inhibitors found in legumes can be at least partially deactivated by thorough soaking and cooking. We'll look at this in more depth later on in this chapter.

The inherent problems legumes may pose need to be weighed against the fact that they are a quite nutritious food. Most beans and lentils are eaten 'whole' – in stark contrast to the refined, nutrient-stripped form we find so many grains in within our diet. Also, again unlike many grains, legumes generally have low GIs and GLs, which has vitally important implications for health and well-being (see Chapter 4 for more details about this).

Making a scientifically based judgement of legumes is difficult, as these foods have not been the subject of much nutritionally focused research. There is, for instance, a dearth of evidence looking at the relationship between legume intake and the conditions heart disease and diabetes. However, their slow sugar-releasing nature would be expected to translate into biochemical benefits that should protect against these conditions.

There is more evidence in the area of cancer, the results of which are very mixed. In one review of 58 studies, 29 reported a decreased risk with higher legume intake whereas 22 reported an increased risk.[27] Overall, the balance of evidence suggests that legumes are unlikely to have an important influence on cancer risk either way.

The intake of legumes and other foods was assessed in a study which attempted to link diet with longevity in Japan, Sweden, Greece and Australia.[28] Of all the foods analysed, the only one that was consistently associated with increased lifespan was legumes. This does not, of course, prove that legumes were the life-extending factor. But the results of this study at least support the notion that beans and lentils have some place in a healthy diet.

Pulses can be used as an accompaniment to a meal (e.g. Puy lentils), or as an addition to salads, stews or soups. Homemade hummus, the main ingredient of which is chickpeas, is another good option. Baked beans, mainly on account of their high sugar and salt content, should be regarded as nutritionally inferior to less-processed forms of pulses.

As with grain-based foods, 'gatherers' tend to do better on pulses than 'hunters'.

Preparing Pulses

As discussed earlier, legumes can contain substances called 'lectins' that may be responsible for food-sensitivity reactions, as well as 'enzyme inhibitors' that can impair digestion. These components can be deactivated, to a large degree, through appropriate preparation and cooking.

As far as preparation is concerned, soaking is the key. If you're intending to cook beans from their dried state, they should first be soaked for several (generally 4–12) hours. The most convenient time to do this is generally overnight. The soaking water should be discarded and the beans should be rinsed before cooking in unsalted water (salt tends to toughen their skins). An alternative to this lengthy preparation time is to buy canned pulses. However, before preparation it is best to rinse them thoroughly as this will help to remove as much added salt and sugar as possible.

Thorough cooking of legumes will not just help to nullify lectins and enzyme inhibitors, but can also reduce the levels of certain starches in beans that can ferment in the gut and cause wind.[29]

Soy Good?

Perhaps one of the most widely eaten beans of all is the soya bean. Actually, the bean itself is hardly, if ever, eaten, but food products prepared from components of the bean are. The oil derived from soya beans finds its way into many processed foods. Also, the protein-rich part of the bean can be spun into a wide range of foods including tofu, soya milk, tempeh and miso. There have been a range of health claims made for soy, including an ability to reduce cholesterol levels and ward off breast cancer and osteoporosis. But is soy really the versatile wonderfood it is so often made out to be?

First of all, we should be aware that despite its widespread use in the diet, soya is actually a relatively new food – soy beans were probably first cultivated no more than 3,000 years ago. Like other legumes, soybeans contain substances that can impair digestion, which can reduce the nutritional value of the foods we eat and enhance the risk of food sensitivities, too. Although these toxic compounds are largely deactivated or removed during the processing of soybeans into products such as tofu, tempeh and miso, there is the risk that at least some of them will remain in the finished product.

Soybeans are also rich in a substance known as 'phytic acid' – a compound which impairs the absorption of a range of minerals including calcium, magnesium, iron and zinc. Phytic acid is also found in grains, but soybeans seem to be especially rich in this anti-nutrient.[30] Unfortunately, cooking does not seem to destroy phytic acid, though levels of this compound can be reduced (though not necessarily eliminated) through the fermentation of soy into foods such as tempeh and miso.

The food industry has contrived to spin soya out into a huge range of processed foods by converting raw soya beans into something known as 'soy protein isolate' (SPI). Production of SPI takes place in factories where a slurry of soy beans is treated with acid and alkali solutions to get the protein to precipitate out. In this process the product can be tainted with the metal aluminium (aluminium exposure has been linked with an increased risk of degeneration of the nervous system and Alzheimer's disease). The resultant protein-rich 'curd' is spray-dried at high temperature to produce a powder. SPI may then be heated and extruded under pressure to make a foodstuff known as 'textured vegetable protein' (TVP). SPI and TVP will often have monosodium glutamate (MSG) added to impart a 'meaty' flavour. Once flavoured, SPI can be shaped into a wide range of foods including meat-substitute products such as vegetarian burgers, sausages and mince.

Versatile SPI may be, but it is actually a very heavily processed food. What are its effects on health? Certain toxins found in soya, including digestion-inhibitors looked at earlier in this chapter, are known to remain in SPI.[31] Animal experiments suggest that eating SPI can lead to a deficiency of a range of nutrients including calcium, magnesium, manganese, copper, iron and zinc.[32] Soy also seems to have the capacity to impair thyroid function, which can lead to diverse symptoms such as weight gain, fatigue and low mood.[33] (For more information on the thyroid and its role in health, see Appendix D.)

And what of the health claims so often made for soya? After all, it is often promoted for its ability to reduce cholesterol levels. This would be a blessing as long as cholesterol-reduction through dietary means had been shown to be beneficial to health – which it hasn't (see Chapter 8 for more on this).

Soya has also been heavily promoted for its breast cancer-protective effects. This proposed benefit has been put down to hormone-like molecules known as phytoestrogens that are found in soya. These are often said to help block the breast cancer-causing potential of the hormone oestrogen in the female body. However, the research results in this area are very mixed, and there is simply no clear evidence supporting the role of dietary phytoestrogens in the prevention of breast cancer.[34]

Also, it is possible that plant compounds that mimic oestrogen may actually have an *adverse* effect on health. It is known, for instance, that high levels of oestrogen have been associated with an increased rate of mental decline associated with ageing. It is interesting, then, that one study has found a significant statistical relationship between the eating of tofu and accelerated brain ageing.[35]

With all this in mind, does soy really deserve its 'superfood' reputation? I don't think so, and moreover I believe the science shows it makes sense not to emphasize soy-based foods in the diet. Forms of soy that seem particularly worth avoiding are SPI and TVP. The best forms of soy are likely to be more natural ones that have also been fermented, such as tempeh, natto and miso.

The Question of Quorn

Another food favourite of vegetarians, vegans or individuals just wanting to eat more 'healthily' is Quorn. The main ingredient in this foodstuff is 'mycoprotein'. What's that? You may well ask. Mycoprotein actually is made from a mould organism ('Fusarium venenatum') found in soil. This organism is multiplied *en masse* in steel containers and then contrived into, among other things, 'burgers', 'sausages' and other meat-substitute foods.

Part of Quorn's healthy image is fostered by references made by its manufacturers to its low-fat and cholesterol-free nature. Well, as we saw in Chapter 8 (Lean Times) this is unlikely to offer any benefits to the body. And besides, even if it did, we need to consider the suitability of the whole food on the body. Cow dung may be fat and cholesterol free, but that doesn't make it a healthy food.

Another tack taken by Quorn's manufacturers is to give its product a natural image by likening it to mushrooms and truffles. According to Professor David Geiser of the Fusarium Research Center at Pennsylvania State University in the US, drawing parallels between the organism used to make Quorn and mushrooms is like 'calling a rat a chicken because both are animals'.[36] And this novel food has been linked with adverse reactions including gastrointestinal complaints.[37]

Like SPI and TVP, Quorn is a highly processed and quite unnatural food. Personally, I don't recommend it at all.

So, Is it Animal or Vegetable?

The evidence suggests that both animal and plant-based 'primal' foods are nutritious and have health-giving properties. Nevertheless, there's generally a thought out there that vegetarian and vegan diets are healthier than more omnivorous ones that contain flesh foods such as meat and fish. Those who espouse vegetarian or vegan eating will often quote the 'evidence' which, we are told, shows that these ways of eating are associated with a significantly reduced risk of heart disease and longer life.

Actually, bearing in mind the fact that our evolutionary diet generally contained quite a lot of meat and that no modern hunter-gatherer societies have been found to be vegetarian, the idea that not eating animal foods is 'healthy' does not make sense. And let's not forget that animal foods, including meat, can supply nutrients that are difficult or impossible to get from a vegetarian or vegan diet. A case in point is vitamin B_{12}. This nutrient is only found in animal products. So if vegans want to avoid running low in this nutrient and its potential consequences (which include anaemia, neurological symptoms and dementia), they must supplement with it. This, of course, strongly suggests that the vegan diet is inadequate on its own to support good health.

Vegetarian and vegan diets are also at risk of being low on protein. This dietary element provides building-blocks (amino acids) that can be reassembled into body components including bone and soft tissues. Research exists which shows that higher levels of protein intake are associated with enhanced height and lean weight in children.[38] And protein, as we learned above, is also important for quelling the appetite.

Amino acids – the building-blocks of protein – come in 22 different types, 10 of which must be supplied by the diet for optimal growth and well-being. The full spectrum of these so-called 'essential amino acids' is found more readily in animal foods than plant fare. Those on a vegan diet will improve their chances of getting enough of these essential amino acids by emphasizing a wide range of foods rich in protein such as beans, lentils, nuts and seeds. These foods are obviously appropriate for vegetarians, who also have the option of finding quality protein in dairy products such as milk, cheese and yoghurt. Unfortunately, these foods are a common cause of food-sensitivity issues (see Chapter 6 and Appendix A for more details about this) and, contrary to popular opinion, do little or nothing to support the health of our bones.

Other deficiencies that may befall vegetarians and vegans include those of iron,[39] zinc,[40] and iodine.[41] Iron deficiency can cause anaemia, but even in the absence of this a low level of iron in the body can cause fatigue and low mood (see the section on iron, page 87). Zinc deficiency may manifest in a variety of ways including lowered immunity and a reduced sense of taste and smell. And iodine is vitally important for the healthy function of the thyroid gland, any failure in which can lead to a range of symptoms such as sensitivity to cold, weight gain, fatigue and depression.

This sort of evidence does seem to take the healthy sheen off vegetarian and vegan diets. So, what about that 'evidence' that shows that vegetarian and vegan eating is better for us?

Studies do exist which appear to show that vegetarians are less likely to succumb to heart disease and tend to live longer, too. However, such studies are what are known as 'epidemiological' in nature, which means that while they can show associations between two factors (in this case, vegetarian eating and better health), they cannot be used to 'prove' that vegetarianism is healthy. This is because the apparent benefits to health may come from other factors associated with vegetarianism, such as a reduced tendency to smoke and healthier exercise habits. These so-called 'confounding factors' need to be taken into consideration in order to make a fair assessment of the relative merits of vegetarian, vegan and non-vegetarian diets.

The most recent research in which potential confounding factors were taken into account was performed by UK-based researchers.[42] In this study, the dietary habits of some 56,000 individuals were assessed, after which they were classified into 'vegetarian' and 'non-vegetarian' categories. In addition, though, the participants' body weight, smoking habits and alcohol consumption were taken into consideration. Once these potential confounding factors were accounted for, there was no difference in death rates between vegetarians and non-vegetarians.

This study also analysed data from two other studies in which attempts had been made to take account of the fact that vegetarians are generally more health-conscious than non-vegetarians. In one of these studies, researchers attempted to counteract any confounding factors by focusing only on individuals who shopped in health-food stores.[43] The idea here is that health-food store shoppers are generally 'health-conscious', whether they are vegetarian or not. This allows a fairer appraisal of the impact of vegetarian or non-vegetarian eating. In this study, the overall risk of death in vegetarians and non-vegetarians was found to be the same.

In the other study, vegetarians were asked to recruit their friends and family into the study.[44] Doing this was thought to help ensure that all individuals in the study were similarly health-conscious. Again, this study found that the death rates for vegetarians and non-vegetarians were the same.[43]

And what of the claim about vegetarian diets being better for the heart? All three of these studies found that rates of heart disease were the same in vegetarian and non-vegetarian groups. So, the plain facts show that, overall, there is no broad health advantage to be gained from eating a vegetarian or vegan diet.

The Bottom Line

- The major 'primal' foods that remain in the modern-day diet include animal foods such as meat, fish and eggs, and plant-based foods such as fruits, vegetables and nuts.

- Meat is a highly nutritious food that is a good source of protein (which, among other things, can help sate the appetite), iron, zinc, B vitamins, carnitine and monounsaturated fat.

- The evidence suggests that unprocessed meats are healthier than processed meats such as salami and bacon.

- Eggs are also a rich source of protein and nutrients such as monounsaturated fat, iron and B_{12}. Their eating does not have a strong link with heart disease.

- Fish and seafood help provide the body with important nutrients like iodine and zinc. Some fish are a good source of the so-called omega-3 fats that have important benefits for the cardiovascular system and brain.

- Fruit and vegetables are rich in nutrients including potentially disease-protective substances known as phytochemicals. Their eating has been associated with a reduced risk of both cardiovascular disease and cancer

- Fruits and vegetables are almost certainly healthier in an organic form. Non-organic fruits and vegetables should be washed prior to consumption.

- Potatoes generally have high glycaemic indices and loads, and tend to be lower in nutritional value than other vegetables.

- Nuts are a highly nutritious food that seem to help protect against heart disease. Eating them does not appear to cause weight gain.

- Beans and lentils, like grains, are a relatively recent addition to the human diet. They may cause problems with food sensitivity and also contain compounds that have an 'anti-nutrient' effect. However, beans and lentils are a good source of protein, liberate sugar slowly into the bloodstream, and can be prepared and cooked in a way that can counteract some of their less healthy properties.

- Soya and Quorn, though often recommended as 'health foods', have a number of properties that make them far from ideal for human consumption.

- In contrast to conventional wisdom, studies show that vegetarian diets are not inherently healthier than more omnivorous ones.

Chapter 10 Fluid Thinking

Until now, this book has been mainly focused on what it means to *eat* a healthy diet. However, healthy nutrition isn't just about what we eat, but also what we *drink*. So in this chapter we shall be taking an in-depth look at the major fluids in the modern-day diet, and examining what effects they have on health. We shall start with water, the most fundamental of fluids, before moving on to other popular beverages such as coffee, tea and alcohol.

Water, Water, Everywhere

The adult human body is about 60 per cent water, and this fact alone suggests that this fluid has an important part to play in health and well-being. Actually, all of our biochemical, physiological and neurological processes depend, to some degree, on water. For instance, water makes up the bulk of our blood volume. If we do not keep ourselves properly topped up with fluid, then this may be reflected in a slightly reduced blood volume and blood pressure. The end result here is that our circulation may fail to deliver oxygen and nutrients to all our tissues and organs with optimal efficiency. The circulation is key to ensuring proper detoxification of the body and elimination of waste through the kidneys. A spot of dehydration might therefore increase the risk of toxic build-up in the body, which is likely to have a negative impact on our health and well-being. Water is also important for nerve transmission in the body. Running low on fluid can therefore have consequences for brain function. Water basically helps all body and brain processes run that much more smoothly. No wonder, then, that while the human body can usually go a few weeks or even months without food, it can only manage a few days without water.

What Are the Benefits of Drinking Water?

Bearing in mind its critical role in the body's most fundamental processes, we should not be too surprised that even relatively mild dehydration can manifest in a myriad of ways. My overwhelming experience in practice is that when individuals become dehydrated, they don't usually feel great. Lethargy is a common manifestation, both of body and mind. Put another way, when individuals who are not in the habit of drinking much water make more of an effort in this area, they almost always feel better for it. Many individuals who get a bit more water into their system find this buoys up their mental and physical energies, often within half an hour or so.

Another quite common consequence of dehydration is headache. One theory about how this happens is that running low on fluid can cause the membranes that cover the brain (called 'meninges') to exert some downward pressure which is sensed as pain. I don't know whether this is true or not. But what I do know is that many individuals with 'mystery' headaches often banish them simply by drinking more water.

And dehydration can cause constipation, too. When the body runs dry, it does its utmost to extract every last drop of water from waste matter in the large colon. The end result can be a bit like a cork stuck in the neck of a wine bottom. Keeping well hydrated is often a crucial tactic in keeping our bowels moving nicely along.

Does Water Have Any Long-term Benefits?

A lack of fluid intake obviously causes the urine to be more concentrated – something that can increase the risk of developing kidney or bladder stones (known as 'urinary calculi'). Research shows that kidney stones are more common in populations where urine volume is low. More importantly, perhaps, studies show that increasing urine volume to about 2–2½ litres each day reduces the risk of kidney stones.[1-4] Anyone wanting to protect themselves from kidney stones would therefore do well to ensure a good fluid intake, and this is particularly important for individuals who have a history of this condition.

There is also some evidence that drinking more water can help keep us free from serious conditions such as cancer and heart disease. One study, for instance, found that increasing fluid intake was associated with a reduced risk of cancer of the bladder.[5] Other research has found a link between increased water consumption and a reduced risk of cancer of the colon.[6] It is not known for certain how water drinking might reduce cancer risk. Although, at the very least, good hydration is likely to dilute and speed the elimination of toxic, cancer-inducing substances within the body, particularly from the bladder and colon.

Water consumption has also been linked with a reduced risk of heart disease. In one study, drinking five or more glasses of water each day, compared to drinking two or fewer, was associated with a 54 and 41 per cent reduced risk in dying from heart disease in men and women respectively.[7]

For optimal health and well-being, the evidence shows it pays to keep topped up with water.

How Much Water Do We Need?

Water is clearly fundamental to health, but how much do we *really* need? Is it true that we need eight (or is it 12) glasses of water each day? Well, there's no doubt in my mind that our needs for water are highly individual and depend on, among other things, our size and shape, the temperature and humidity in our environment, the amount of exercise we take and our capacity for sweating. What this means is that it's very difficult to make blanket recommendations about water intake which may be too much for some people while being not enough for others.

Because of this, I encourage individuals to 'tune in to' their body and be alert for signs of their state of hydration. Thirst is not a good sign, as by the time the body is thirsty it is often quite dehydrated indeed. A good gauge, though, to the state of our hydration is the colour of our urine.[8] Essentially, the paler in colour our urine, the better our state of hydration. The aim is to keep our urine colour pale yellow throughout the day. If urine colour strays into darker tones, particularly if this is accompanied by a noticeable smell, then it's time to step up our water intake. Most individuals, most of the time, need to drink in the order of 2–3 litres of water each day to maintain a good state of hydration.

Keep Water by You

For many people, the idea of drinking 2 or 3 litres of water a day seems quite a feat. The one big piece of advice I have about getting plenty of water into the body each day is this – *keep water by you*. I know this is obvious, but you can't drink water from a bottle in the fridge or a water cooler down the end of the corridor *unless* you are by that source of water or you bring the water to you. For this reason, I suggest keeping water readily to hand.

If you're doing the gardening, keep a bottle of water with you. Put a bottle of water on your desk at work, and make sure there is water available in meetings. Put a half-litre bottle of water in the car and carry one in your handbag or briefcase when you are out and about. My experience with clients has led me to conclude that if we keep water by us we generally get through decent quantities of the stuff, but if we don't – we *won't*.

Can I Drink Too Much Water?

Excessive drinking of water can, in theory, cause a lowering of sodium levels in the body (the medical term for which is 'hyponatraemia'), which can lead to swelling of the brain (cerebral oedema) with potentially fatal consequences. There is no risk of this in individuals drinking even several litres of water each day, as long as this is consumed over the course of the day and not all at once.

One group of individuals who are at some risk of water overload are those engaged in endurance exercise such as marathon running. Here, sodium losses through sweating coupled with very high intake of water over several hours can lead to hyponatraemia and the complications this may bring. The risk of this is higher in warm or hot weather, where sweating and water intake are likely to be greater.

The risk of 'water intoxication' during endurance exercise is very small but does exist. Being mindful of the need for adequate but not excessive water intake during endurance exercise will help protect against water intoxication, as will the consumption of 'electrolyte' drinks that contain sodium.

What Form of Water?

Most of us can get water straight from the tap. The thinking out there is that bottled water is better for us. The municipal water companies tell us this is nonsense. So, what's the truth?

Tap Water

Do you ever really give any thought to where your tap water comes from? The precise original source will vary from location to location, but for most of us what comes out of our taps is sanitized water that comes from water that's already made its way through dishwashers, washing machines, baths and showers.

For water to be made 'fit to drink' it is first allowed to sit so that some of the impurities can sediment out. After this, the water is treated chemically (generally with aluminium) to encourage the sedimentation of some of the lighter impurities in the water. Next the water is filtered, after which it is disinfected. Disinfection generally involves chlorine, although ozone and ultraviolet light radiation are other more expensive options. And then after all of that, water comes down pipes and into our homes.

All this processing is designed to make the look and taste of water acceptable to us, and ensure that it does not contain any nasty bugs. However, the processing of water can taint it with substances that might not be the best for the body. Take chlorine, for instance. This disinfectant is what is known as an 'oxidizing' agent, which means it can induce chemical changes which, at least in theory, could increase cancer risk. Water may also contain compounds that are by-products of the chlorination process known as 'trihalomethanes', which are also thought to have cancer-inducing potential.

A review of 10 studies which examined the link between chlorine and its by-products found that exposure to these chemicals was associated with a 21 and 38 per cent increased risk of bladder and rectal cancers respectively.[9] Another study found that exposure to chlorine or trihalomethanes was associated with an increased risk of brain tumours.[10] These associations do not prove that tap water causes cancer. However, the fact that these associations exist, coupled with a plausible mechanism by which the compounds in tap water might cause cancer, should, I think, give us some cause for concern.

And what of aluminium, which is used to take particulate matter out of water? There is some concern that this metal has some role to play in Alzheimer's disease.[11] While the evidence is not clear-cut, it suggests that aluminium exposure through drinking water is associated with an increased risk of this condition.

Another potential additive in tap water is fluoride. This substance is added to the water in some countries because it is said to protect teeth from decay. The most comprehensive study to look at this association – often referred to as the 'York study' – did indeed confirm this to be the case.[12] However, the York study also found that the protection offered by fluoride is actually far lower than previously thought: just one in six people drinking fluoridated water benefits from this practice. However, drinking fluoridated water was also found to cause 'dental fluorosis' (a condition in which the teeth become mottled due to excess fluoride) in almost half of individuals drinking fluoridated water. One might question the wisdom of preventing dental disease in one in six, while at the same time *causing* dental disease in one in two.

Also, because dental fluorosis is a sign of fluoride toxicity, could it be that fluoride ingestion might also lead to more sinister health effects deeper inside the body? There is at least some evidence which suggests, for instance, that fluoride exposure may increase the risk of bone fracture. Some research also suggests that fluoride may have toxic effects on many parts of the body including the brain and thyroid gland. More information about these and other potential hazards of fluoride can be found at www.fluoridealert.org.

What Can Be Done to Improve Tap Water Quality?
Because of the chemical constituents so often found in tap water, my advice is to avoid it, at least straight from the tap. However, tap water can be filtered in a way that will reduce some of its potentially harmful qualities. A simple and relatively inexpensive way to do this is to use a jug which has an integrated filter. These filters help to get rid of much of the chlorine and other chemicals that may be in your tap water, but will allow most of the healthy minerals in water (see below) to get through. It is important to remember to change the filter frequently (most are good for 50–200 litres of water).

A step up from jug filters are filters which are plumbed into the water supply. These generally contain carbon filters, though some also include fine clay particles to help filter out bacteria. These are more expensive than the jug filters (expect to pay about £200) and the cartridges do need replacing (usually annually). However, they are very convenient and generally do a very good job.

Another form of 'in-house' water purification is known as the 'reverse osmosis system'. This is good for removing impurities including bacteria, but also removes whatever minerals the water may contain. The systems are on the expensive side, quite costly to run, and discard about 80 per cent of the water they treat. For these reasons, I prefer the plumbed-in filters.

Mineral Water

Another option open to those wanting to get all of the potential benefits of water with few or none of the potential hazards is to drink mineral water. According to European law, mineral waters must emerge from the ground in a state fit to drink, and must be bottled at source. The water must also be protected from pollution to ensure its purity. All this means that the potential contamination issues with tap water (relating to substances such as chlorine, trihalomethanes, aluminium and fluoride) just don't apply.

The big downside to bottled water (apart from the inconvenience factor and cost) relates to its impact on the environment. In an increasingly polluted world, and one where there is growing awareness about the need to reduce our 'carbon footprint' as much as possible, it becomes harder and harder to justify drinking mineral waters that hail from foreign parts. Because of these concerns, I recommend drinking mineral water in its country of origin.

Still or Sparkling?

Before we go anywhere with this, let me say that my personal belief is that whether one drinks sparkling or still water is a marginal issue. Compared to the question of, say, whether to drink diet cola or mineral water, the one regarding whether it is better to drink still or sparkling mineral water pales into insignificance. While there is a general thought out there that still is healthier than sparkling, one study found that drinking sparkling water brought about changes in the bloodstreams of women which would be expected to reduce the risk of heart disease more than drinking still water.[13] On the other hand, carbonated water can increase the risk of problems like indigestion and erosion of tooth enamel. My advice is to drink the one you like: this may help you drink more, and the positive effects of this are likely to outweigh any potential disadvantages of drinking a specific type of water. Individuals opting for sparkling water might consider drinking this through a straw, which will reduce the risk of dental erosion.

Does It Have to Be Water?

Not everything we eat or drink should be determined by its likely effects on our health and well-being. Some of us may be inclined to consume things that we believe are not the best thing for us because we *like* them. Besides, some people don't like drinking water, or just like a bit of variety. So, what beverages offer an alternative to water, and what effects do they have on the body?

Fruit Juice

Fruit juices are often seen as healthy drinks that are roughly equivalent to whole fruit. However, in the juicing of a fruit many nutritious elements, in particular its fibre and also a proportion of its nutrients, are left behind. Fruit juice also contains a hefty dose of the sugar fructose. While this sugar is traditionally thought of as quite healthy, there is evidence that it is really no better than other forms of sugar such as sucrose (table sugar) and, in excessive quantities, may give rise to problems including weight gain and diabetes[14] (see page 44).

Most commercially available juices are dehydrated and then reconstituted with water – processing which undoubtedly reduces their nutritional value, too. The best fruit juices are those that are freshly squeezed. Home-made is best, though diluting these with water (about half and half) is a good idea. It helps to temper their 'sugariness' by diluting the fructose and other sugars in them. Commercially available 'freshly squeezed' juices are obviously not as 'fresh' as home prepared, and are also flash-pasteurized (two factors that are likely to reflect on their nutrient content), but are generally a good second best to home-made stuff. Further down in the pecking order is the cartoned stuff, with the juices made of concentrate – as is the case with most of them – being the worst of the lot.

Another option for fruit-based drinks is the 'smoothie'. These drinks are generally better than juices, as many of them contain whole fruit mashed up, rather than juiced fruit. Like freshly squeezed juices these are pasteurized, but almost certainly retain many beneficial nutritional qualities. Look at the ingredients label – the best smoothies list fruit or fruit juice, and nothing else. Of course, you could always make your own.

One final thing: Do not be tempted to confuse fruit 'juice' with fruit 'drink'. Products labelled 'fruit drink' need only to contain as little as 5 per cent fruit juice by law, and often contain a lot of unwanted additives besides. In particular, many contain artificial sweeteners. Fruit drinks are to be avoided, as is anything labelled 'fruit-flavoured' – these do not need to contain *any* fruit at all.

Diluted fruit juices and smoothies tend to suit 'gatherers' best, though I do recommend that they are consumed in limited amounts only. 'Hunters' tend not to do well on such drinks at all.

Herbal and Fruit Teas

Herbal and fruit teas may have some therapeutic benefit for the body. Fennel and peppermint, for instance, may aid digestion, while chamomile can aid restful sleep. I reckon, from a hydration perspective, herbal and fruit teas are a decent swap for water. What about harder stuff?

Tea

Tea comes in two main forms – black and green. Basically, black tea is made from allowing green tea to undergo oxidation. Both black and green tea contain caffeine and other stimulants, as well as disease-protective compounds known as 'polyphenols' that have 'antioxidant' activity. This means they have the capacity to neutralize the effects of damaging, disease-causing molecules called 'free radicals'. In general terms, green tea contains less caffeine and has more antioxidant capacity than black tea.

Black Tea and Health

There is quite a lot of research which links black tea consumption with a reduced risk of heart disease. Recently, a review in the *European Journal of Clinical Nutrition* confirmed this association. Drinking 3 or more cups of black tea seems to be what is required to get this benefit.[15] The review also found that, despite the fact that tea contains some caffeine and other substances that have a diuretic effect (meaning they stimulate urine production), drinking tea did not generally cause dehydration in the body.

Some people seem to turn to tea at times of stress or shock. I've always thought that this was culturally based. Recent evidence has caused me to review this belief, however: researchers in London, UK, have found that tea drinking helps reduce levels of stress hormones after an emotionally challenging event.[16] It seems that there might be some basis for using a cup of tea to help calm our nerves.

Green Tea and Health

Like black tea, green tea is rich in polyphenols, and this may help to explain why research has linked green tea consumption with a reduced risk of heart disease.[17] One of the polyphenols found in green tea goes by the name of 'epigallocatechin gallate' (EGCG). This compound has been found to have a number of cancer-protective actions in the body, including an ability to help in the deactivation of cancer-causing chemicals (carcinogens). There is evidence to suggest that regular consumption of green tea is associated with a reduced risk of some forms of cancer.[18]

Coffee

Coffee has a reputation as the devil's brew. This drink's naturally high caffeine nature often gives it the image of a beverage that can induce all sorts of issues including raised blood pressure, palpitations and insomnia. Caffeine and other stimulants found in coffee can be a problem in excess (see the section entitled Caffeine and Health, below), but does coffee really deserve the unhealthy reputation it seems to have acquired? The evidence suggests not.

To start with, coffee is very rich in 'antioxidant' substances including polyphenols. The drinking of coffee is actually very consistently associated with a reduced risk of diabetes[19] and metabolic syndrome[20] (see Chapter 4 for more on this condition). Other research has found coffee drinking associated with a reduced risk of cardiovascular disease in women.[21] This study actually found that women drinking 1–3 cups of coffee a day were 24 per cent less likely to die from cardiovascular disease. In another study, coffee consumption was associated with a reduced overall risk of death in individuals with Type 2 diabetes.[22]

The idea that tea and coffee might be beneficial to health may not seem to make sense from an evolutionary perspective. After all, these beverages are relatively recent additions to the diet. However, the main constituent of these drinks is *water*. Of course, that won't always guarantee that a beverage is healthy: the prime constituent of a solution of arsenic and cyanide is also water, but I wouldn't recommend drinking it! But let's not forget that coffee comes from a bean and tea from a leaf. When analysed chemically, both turn out to be rich in health-promoting substances (including the polyphenols mentioned above). When such substances are infused into some hot water, it's perhaps not that surprising that the resulting beverages turn out to have benefits for health.

Caffeine and Health

While coffee and tea are broadly beneficial to health, they also contain caffeine and other stimulants that, in excess, can trigger everything from anxiety to heart rhythm irregularities to sleeplessness. So, while some of your favourite brew may be OK, it's possible to get too much of it, too. How much is too much is a highly individual affair, though. The reason for this relates to the fact that caffeine is metabolized (and rendered inactive) in the liver through a process known as 'acetylation'. And some people can do this more efficiently than others.

Brisk metabolizers of caffeine find they tend not to get much of a 'boost' from caffeine, and as a result are not particularly prone to caffeine addiction. As a general rule, rapid metabolizers of caffeine will also find that caffeine tends not to disrupt their sleep. Slower metabolizers, on the other hand, do tend to get a 'kick' from caffeine, and can often easily find themselves depending on it a bit. Slow metabolizers will also be prone to sleep-disruption should they consume too much caffeine. These individuals, obviously, need to be a bit more careful with their caffeine consumption.

In practice, I find that 'gatherers' tend to do better on caffeine than 'hunters'.

One simple way to avoid drinking too much coffee or tea is to ensure that when you do drink it, you make sure it's good stuff. All that rubbishy instant coffee and machine-vended varieties which can make up the bulk of our intake can usually be dispensed with without being missed. Making your own espresso or cafetière coffee, brewing a nice pot of tea or getting a decent brew from a coffee shop ensures that whatever coffee and tea you consume may be enjoyed and even savoured. The time and effort spent in opting for quality coffee or tea tends to put an automatic ceiling on the amount that is consumed. Concentrating on quality will generally take care of any issues with regard to quantity.

Another option for those keen not to overdo the caffeine is to opt for decaf. Decaffeination processes generally involve chemical solvents that are best avoided. More natural, and preferred, forms of decaffeination use water (also known as the 'Swiss' method) or carbon dioxide. Some scrutinizing of labels is required to find appropriate brands.

Alcohol

For as long as I can remember, moderate alcohol consumption has been touted as 'healthy'. Red wine, in particular, we are told has benefits for the heart. Men and women are told they can benefit from drinking up to 21 and 14 units (a unit is equivalent to a small glass of wine) respectively per week. This advice is based on the results of research which shows that moderate drinkers are at a reduced risk of heart disease compared to those who don't drink at all.

When we take a closer look at the evidence regarding alcohol and health, we see that the studies on which current recommendations are based leave quite a lot to be desired. In these studies, individuals in the teetotal group may include, for instance, reformed alcoholics. As alcoholism is likely to lead to long-term damage to the heart, this might artificially push up the heart disease rates seen in teetotal groups. Also, one reason why people may be abstaining from drink is that they have been diagnosed with heart disease and therefore have been advised to cut out alcohol or have decided for themselves to take this step. Basically, this can bias the results of the studies and make it seem that abstaining from alcohol is not as healthy as it might be in reality.

Another major flaw of the oft-quoted alcohol research is that it has often focused on heart disease only. This is an important condition, but it accounts for only about a quarter of deaths. What about the other three-quarters? As it happens, alcohol is known to increase the risk of other conditions that can prove fatal, including liver disease and several forms of cancer. Therefore, to make a decent judgement of the effects of alcohol on health we shouldn't really be focusing only on heart disease deaths, but overall risk of death (also known as 'funeral rates').

When researchers have focused on overall mortality, a slightly different picture from the 'healthy tipple' image of alcohol emerges. One study found that in women up to the age of 54 and men up to the age of 34, the optimal amount of alcohol to drink was none at all.[23] In this study, there seemed to be some benefits of alcohol consumption later in life. Optimal intakes of alcohol for men and women over the age of 65 were 8 units and 3 units respectively a *week*. These levels of alcohol consumption are far lower than generally recommended. As a drinker myself, I take no satisfaction in imparting this news, but it seems the 'benefits' of drinking alcohol have been somewhat overstated.

One tactic for coping with this none-too-cheery news is simply to balance alcohol with water. For instance, for each glass of wine you drink, drink one of water. This will often reduce the amount of alcohol drunk in the long term – there's only so much room in the stomach, after all. It also literally dilutes any damage the alcohol may do. Plus, the additional water is health-giving, right? So, by balancing alcohol with water we do ourselves and our bodies a real favour.

Is Red Wine Any Better?

Red wine, more than any other form of alcohol, has been recommended as 'healthy'. Much scientific focus has been put on a constituent of red grapes known as resveratrol, the actions of which in the body would help to explain red wine's proposed benefits for the heart.

However, a close look at the evidence reveals that wine drinkers, compared to those who generally choose other forms of alcohol, like beer and spirits, tend to eat healthier diets and smoke less, too.[24-6] It seems it's not the red wine *per se*, but these other factors associated with drinking it that account for its apparent 'benefits'.

The Bottom Line

• Water plays an important role in physiological and neurological processes in the body and brain.

• In the short term, dehydration can lead to symptoms such as mental and physical lethargy, headaches and constipation.

• In the long term, low water intake has been associated with an increased risk of kidney stones, cancer and heart disease.

• Tap water consumption is linked with adverse effects on health including an increased risk of some forms of cancer.

• Before consumption, tap water should be filtered. Mineral water is another option, though for environmental reasons this is best drunk in its country of origin.

• Fruit juice is very sugary and has limited nutritional value. Ideally, it should be freshly squeezed and diluted with water prior to consumption.

• Herbal and fruit teas make a healthy alternative to water.

• Tea consumption is linked with a reduced risk of cardiovascular disease, and green tea consumption may help reduce cancer risk.

• Coffee consumption is linked with a reduced risk of chronic disease, especially diabetes.

- Caffeine in tea and coffee can have adverse effects on health, though the ability to tolerate caffeine varies from individual to individual. Generally speaking, 'gatherers' tolerate caffeine the best.

- The health 'benefits' of alcohol seem to have been overstated. Balancing alcohol with water is very likely to reduce the negative impact alcohol may have on health.

Chapter 11 **Graze, Don't Gorge**

So far, this book has focused on *what* we should eat for optimal health and well-being. In this chapter we're going to turn our attention to *when* we should eat it. This is because our pattern of eating can influence the efficiency and balance of basic biochemical processes that affect weight and other aspects of health. And regular eating can be vitally important for keeping our appetite in check and stopping it running riot. Counter-intuitive though it may sound, for some individuals looking for improved body weight and well-being, the secret can be not to eat less, but *more*.

Frequent Feeding and Biochemical Balance

In Chapter 4 we explored the importance of ensuring stability in the levels of both sugar and insulin in the body. In the short term, this can help ensure we have consistent levels of mental and physical energy, sleep soundly through the night, and protect ourselves from sudden urges to eat sugar-charged foods such as chocolate and biscuits. In the long term, regulating insulin levels in the body can help protect us from weight gain (particularly around the middle of the body), diabetes, heart disease and, to put it bluntly, death.

Now imagine a scenario where, say, you skip breakfast, eat an inadequate lunch, and then go on, almost inevitably, to polish off a plateful (or two platefuls) of pasta in the evening. Imagine what this might do to blood-sugar and insulin levels at the end of the day, especially if the pasta somehow doesn't quite 'hit the spot' and you find yourself mysteriously drawn to the ice cream tub or biscuit tin sometime later.

To ensure good balance in blood sugar and insulin, it makes sense to eat *regularly*. Perhaps not surprisingly, studies have found that consistent eating is associated with reduced levels of the hormone insulin.[1,2] The implications of this are obviously profound for our long-term health.

Another reason why regularity in eating is important has to do with its ability to control stress hormones in the body. Basically, when we go for long periods of time without eating, the body attempts to fuel itself by mobilizing glucose and other substances from internal stores. Such feeding of the system requires the secretion of 'stress' hormones such as cortisol.

This is important because, while cortisol is essential to life, it can also have a number of detrimental effects in the long term – including an ability to impair insulin's action in the body. It can also enhance the breakdown of bone and muscle in the body. An excess of cortisol may therefore add up to an increased risk of osteoporosis, weight gain and diabetes in the long term. Happily, regular eating has been associated with lower levels of cortisol,[3] which is something we would expect to have favourable effects on health in the long term.

Keeping the Fire Alive

One effect of eating that is very rarely mentioned in relation to weight control is something known as the 'thermogenic effect of food' or 'TEF'. Essentially, the TEF is the little lift in the metabolism that comes after eating. You can think of it a bit like the increase in light and heat you get from a fire after putting some dry wood on it. The TEF may have important implications for weight control because, in theory at least, regular eating may help to maintain the body's metabolism better than more infrequent feeding. A metabolic boost can obviously be a huge boon for those of us who are keen to shed pounds.

The effect of eating patterns on the TEF was tested in a study of women.[4] For two weeks, the women taking part in this research were asked to eat their normal diet, but to consume this as six discrete meals each day. During another two-week spell, the women once again consumed their normal diet, but this time this was divided up into between three and nine portions during the day. The precise number of portions was prescribed by the researchers to ensure that the average number of daily meals or snacks was six (the same number of feeds taken during the other phase of the study). The design of this study enabled the researchers to assess what, if any, advantages regularity in food intake has over more chaotic consumption.

Compared to the irregular eating pattern, regular consumption of food was found to bring a significant rise in the TEF. This study, like others, also found that more consistent consumption of food was associated with lower levels of the hormone insulin. And significantly, the individuals reported eating *less* when eating to a consistent pattern. The findings of this study suggest that regular, frequent eating may assist weight loss in the long term.

Feeding Frequency and Appetite Control

Bearing in mind the dietary restraint that is the cornerstone of weight-management advice, it's perhaps not surprising that many individuals believe that it is only by going hungry that they induce the caloric deficit 'necessary' to lose weight. The fundamental problem here is that, as you may already know, hunger can make it extremely difficult to eat a healthy diet, especially in the long term. For instance, it is not uncommon for individuals who eschew food between meals to simply eat more at meal time. Going hungry can not only increase the amount consumed at a meal, but *what* is eaten. Basically, a roaring appetite can make it nigh on impossible to make the right choice about *what* we eat, and *how much* we eat of it.

Experience shows that individuals eating more regularly tend to get less hungry and find it much easier to exercise restraint as a result. In one study, the effect of different eating patterns on subsequent eating was tested in a group of overweight men.[5] The study participants were fed a set meal, and five hours later were asked to eat freely from a buffet. At another time, the same men were given a fifth of the set meal each hour, before being presented with the same food free-for-all. On both occasions, the researchers measured the number of calories consumed at the buffet. Compared to the single meal, frequent feeding was associated with a reduction in calorie intake of more than a quarter.

Regular Eating Helps Prevent Overeating at Night, Too

Another effect of inadequate or infrequent eating during the day can be a tendency to overeat at night. Many people who find that they can 'get by' on relatively slim pickings for long periods during the waking day can often find that this comes back to bite them in the evening. This may manifest as an overwhelming urge for big or second helpings. Though even then, many will find themselves drawn to still more food in the form of, say, cheese, crackers, ice cream or chocolate.

This phenomenon was studied formally in a piece of research published in the *Journal of Nutrition*.[6] In this study, the diet diaries of almost 800 men and women were examined. Their food and calorific intake was assessed for each of five 4-hour periods stretching from 6 a.m. to 2 a.m. the following day. The results of this study showed that those who had consumed the bulk of their food near the end of the day ate, on average, significantly more calories than individuals who ate more substantial amounts of food early on.

This study, however, did more than just give some scientific credence to the experience of so many who have employed starvation tactics in an effort to lose weight. It also helped to explain what the basis for the late-in-the-day overeating may be. In addition to assessing food intake over the course of each day, the researchers also calculated how effective each meal was at sating the appetite. The so-called 'satiety index' of each meal was calculated by dividing the number of calories it contained into the time that elapsed before another meal or snack was eaten. Interestingly, compared to breakfast and lunch, food eaten in the evening was found to be significantly less likely to satisfy.

Snacking and Weight

Far from being a recipe for weight gain, there is plenty of reason to believe that regular eating might be a useful tactic for those looking to lose weight. There is even some evidence to support this in the form of a study which showed that the more regularly men ate, the lower their body weight and fatness tended to be.[7] This association remained even after accounting for other factors that might help explain it such as physical activity, smoking habits and overall food intake. In another study, individuals eating five or more times a day, compared to those eating three or fewer times each day, were half as likely to be overweight.[8]

Are There Any Other Benefits to Frequent Feeding?

If regular eating helps to stabilize insulin levels, then grazing would be expected to reduce the risk of other conditions associated with insulin excess, such as diabetes and heart disease. In the last study mentioned above,[9] the relationship between meal frequency and risk of diabetes was assessed by measuring something known as 'glucose tolerance' (low glucose tolerance is a risk factor for diabetes). The researchers were unable to look at the risk of diabetes itself, as individuals suffering from this condition were excluded from the study. The results of the study showed that individuals eating five or more times a day, compared to those eating three or fewer times each day, were half as likely to suffer from glucose intolerance.

In another study, meal timing and risk of heart disease were assessed.[10] Individuals eating five or more times a day, compared to those eating three or fewer times each day, were found to be at a significantly reduced risk of heart disease. Frequent eating was associated with a reduction in risk of about a third.

The suggestion here is that, as far as weight loss and general health are concerned, it's better to graze than to gorge.

How Often Should I Eat?

How often someone needs to eat to control appetite and support health varies quite a lot between individuals. My experience in practice is that 'gatherers' can usually get by on three meals a day, with little or nothing in between. If they do feel the need to eat between meals, often something light like a piece of fruit will do the trick and tide them over nicely.

On the other hand, generally speaking, 'hunters' need to eat more frequently. 'Hunters' tend to be hungry people, and therefore in addition to their three meals, often also require snacks in between to keep hunger at bay. In contrast to the 'gatherers', 'hunters' tend not to do well on fruit as a snack, and generally find that it won't really 'touch the sides'. Fattier, more protein-rich snacks such as nuts and seeds tend to suit 'hunters' better.

The Bottom Line

- While eating between meals is generally advised against, there are several reasons why it might actually help enhance health and weight loss.

- Regular eating can help reduce insulin and cortisol levels, two things that would be expected to help reduce the risk of conditions such as obesity and diabetes.

- Regular eating may help maintain the body's metabolism.

- Regular eating helps appetite control, and can therefore assist healthy eating.

- Regular eating and a good intake of food earlier on in the day help to prevent overeating in the evening.

- Regular eating is actually associated with a reduced risk of overweight and obesity, glucose intolerance (a risk factor for diabetes) and heart disease.

- 'Gatherers' will often be able to get by on three meals a day, perhaps with an occasional piece of fruit in between.

- 'Hunters' tend to need to eat very regularly, and find that they require fatty, protein-rich snacks such as nuts to properly satisfy their appetite.

Chapter 12 One Man's Meat ...

In the preceding chapters we have explored what really constitutes a healthy diet. What we've discovered is that it's essentially a diet based on 'primal' foods such as meat, fish, seafood, fruits, vegetables, nuts and seeds. In addition, some carefully chosen dairy products (e.g. butter, yoghurt) and grains (e.g. oats, brown rice, whole rye bread) may also have some place in the diet, along with some appropriately prepared pulses.

While we have been able to draw some broad conclusions about the foods that form the basis of a 'healthy' diet from our ancient past, we also know from experience that our response to specific foods is an individual affair. In the Introduction to this book we looked at how some people have the capacity to thrive on a relatively low-fat, plant-based diet, while others lose weight and feel great on a diet rich in fatty, animal-derived foods.

What this means is that for optimal health and well-being, we need to discover the diet that meets our individual nutritional needs – and that's what *The True You Diet* is all about. In this chapter we're going to examine the evidence for variation in our internal make-up. Here, we'll see why it is that one man's meat really can be another's poison.

The Theory of Nutritional Individuality

In the first chapter of this book (What on Earth Did We Eat?) we looked at what constituted our evolutionary diet, as well as the foods found in more modern 'hunter-gatherer' diets. We learned that there was really no one 'primal diet'. While our ancient diet was made up of natural, unprocessed foods derived from both animals and plants, the relative amounts of foods varied considerably, according to factors such as climate and food availability.

For those of our ancient ancestors living in relatively cold, sometimes harsh climates, plant matter will have been in relatively short supply. In all likelihood, ancestors from such parts would have had no choice but to hunt and eat animal foods such as meat and/or fish. On the other hand, in warmer climates where vegetation was abundant, it may well have been possible for our ancestors to gather and subsist on a diet much richer in plant foods.

As we first explored in the Introduction to this book, the process of evolution means that some of our ancestors would have benefited from becoming adapted to a relatively animal-food-based, fat-rich diet, while others may have enjoyed a distinct advantage by being better suited to a diet richer in plant foods and lower in fat. Still others, of course, may have been adapted to a diet that fell somewhere in between these two extremes. In other words, the genetic adaptation of our ancestors will have marked them out, broadly speaking, as 'hunters', 'gatherers', or 'hunter-gatherers'.

But Do These Different 'Types' Exist Today?

The slow, creeping nature of our genetic material suggests that, at least in theory, these different 'types' of individuals should exist to this day. There is certainly abundant anecdotal evidence that this is indeed the case. Some individuals seem to do very well on a 'low-carb', relatively fatty diet. On the other hand, others find this way of eating simply does not work for them, while a 'lighter' diet lower in fat does. As we learned in the Introduction, research supports these anecdotal experiences. Just to recap, in one study individuals on a low-carb regime saw weight loss in excess of 20kg (equivalent to some 3 stones), while others lost virtually nothing. Then again, the low-fat regime brought spectacular weight loss for some, while being thoroughly ineffective for others.[1] Both experience and the scientific evidence show that what represents a healthy diet varies considerably between individuals.

The Science Behind *The True You Diet*

In recent years, scientists have begun to offer insight into the specifics of how and why our biochemical workings and nutritional needs vary from person to person. To understand this variation, we need first to know the basics of how the body turns food into energy.

All cells in the body (other than the red blood cells) contain tiny 'powerhouses' known as 'mitochondria'. It is in these miniature 'engines' that food is converted into energy. While the processes that make energy from food are complex, for our purposes the most important thing to know is that the mitochondria are fuelled by two major dietary components:

1. Sugar
Actually, glucose, which comes mainly from carbohydrate-rich foods containing sugar and/or starch. Glucose can also be converted from other food elements such as amino acids (the building-blocks of protein) and fat.

2. Fat
This is mainly derived from fat in the diet, though some also comes from fat that has been made within the body by the liver and fat cells.

While both sugar and fat contribute to the fuelling of the body, the relative 'mix' that the body uses to create energy varies between individuals. We know this because the amounts of sugar and fat burned in the body can be measured by analysing the amount of oxygen an individual uses and comparing that with the amount of carbon dioxide released. This comparison allows scientists to calculate what is known as someone's 'respiratory quotient'. This measure provides information about the relative amounts of sugar and fat burned by that individual.

Respiratory quotients vary between 0.7 and 1.0. In theory, if an individual were to burn nothing but sugar, their respiratory quotient would be 1.0. Someone metabolizing nothing but fat would have a respiratory quotient of 0.7. The relative amounts of sugar and fat burned by an individual will dictate where on the spectrum their respiratory quotient lies. Those individuals with high respiratory quotients (near 1.0) tend to use a fuel mix that is relatively rich in sugar and low in fat, while those with low respiratory quotients (nearer 0.7) tend to burn relatively large quantities of fat in comparison to sugar.

If we look back to our past we can see how this might have come about: one could imagine that 'hunters' in the course of our evolution would end up, relatively speaking, being efficient metabolizers of fat, while 'gatherers' would have metabolisms better adapted to the sugar coming ostensibly from carbohydrates.

Perhaps the first person in the modern age to recognize the individual variation in the rate at which foods are metabolized in the body was an American psychologist by the name of Dr George Watson. In 1972 Dr Watson published a book entitled *Nutrition and Your Mind*. In it, the author describes his observation that different people burn fuel in the body at different rates, and how this influences mental functioning. He also describes his approach to treating psychological symptoms using individualized diets and nutritional support. In certain circles George Watson is considered one of the grandfathers of a branch of individualized nutrition often referred to as 'metabolic typing' – essentially, the prescription of diets based on an individual's specific metabolic attributes.

In more recent times scientists have studied individuals with what appear to be quite different metabolic processes. Some of this research has focused on individuals who have different respiratory quotients. Studies have found, for instance, that individuals with relatively high respiratory quotients (relatively slow metabolizers of fat) are more likely to gain weight[2] and are more likely to regain weight after losing it[3,4] compared to those with low respiratory quotients (relatively fast metabolizers of fat).

Scientists have even begun to elucidate what it is about the biochemistry of individuals that accounts for these observations. There is evidence, for instance, that individuals with high respiratory quotients tend to be low in an enzyme called 'lipoprotein lipase'[5] which has a role in breaking down fat in the body, which is a prerequisite for it to be metabolized in the body. Another enzyme important for the metabolism of fat is 'beta-hydroxyl acyl Co A dehydrogenase'. Those with higher respiratory quotients have generally lower levels of this substance, too.[6] It's just these sorts of differences that require nutritional approaches to be tailored to the individual.

What Other Characteristics for the Different Types Have Been Found?

Panning out from the intricacies of our inner workings, scientists have also put some focus on other characteristics of individuals of different types. In particular, there has been recognition that some individuals seem to be able to eat a lot of fat but tend not to put on weight, while others are prone to weight problems should they eat too much fat. These two 'types' of people represent the two ends of a spectrum which correspond to 'hunters' and 'gatherers' respectively. Scientists have noted that the individuals who appear to metabolize fat quite efficiently tend to eat more fat than those who don't (we shall explore this later on).

In one study, the metabolisms of 'hunters' and 'gatherers' were compared.[7] In this study, 'hunters' were found to consume 44 per cent of their calories from fat, while for 'gatherers' this figure was 32 per cent. Compared to the 'gatherers', the 'hunters' had lower respiratory quotients, which means they were better metabolizers of fat, as we'd expect. In addition, though, they were also found to have higher resting metabolic rates, giving them a generally better ability to metabolize food and lower propensity to gain weight. 'Hunters' also had higher pulse rates than 'gatherers'.

In addition, when the individuals were fed a fat-rich diet, the 'hunters' saw a drop in their respiratory quotient, suggesting their body was adapting in the short term in order to metabolize this additional fat. On the other hand, this adjustment was not seen in the 'gatherers'.

This is not the only evidence that has found important differences in individuals' physiological characteristics that may impact on body weight. In one piece of research, the metabolisms of individuals of what was deemed a healthy weight were compared to those of overweight individuals.[8] Those of normal weight were found to have higher metabolic rates, and were more efficient metabolizers of fat, too. The researchers involved in this study also measured the increase in metabolism that comes after eating food – known as the 'thermogenic effect of food' or 'TEF'. The TEF was found to be lower in the overweight individuals compared to those of normal weight.

In another study, lean and overweight individuals were fed a high-carbo-hydrate, low-fat meal to see what effect it had on their physiology.[9] After this meal there was a tendency for overweight individuals, compared to the lean study subjects, to burn fat less effectively and manufacture more fat within the body.

So, it seems that there are several lines of evidence that 'hunters' have brisker metabolisms than 'gatherers'. This makes sense when you consider that 'hunters' are likely to have evolved largely in colder climates. A faster metabolism would be a distinct advantage here as it would help in the generation of heat required to maintain body temperature.

A faster metabolism means that food is going to get burned more quickly, which means a generally greater need for food. In one study, the appetites of individuals eating higher-fat ('hunter') and lower-fat ('gatherer') diets were compared.[10] The individuals were fed a set meal, after which their intake of other foods over the next few hours was measured. Compared to the 'gatherers', the 'hunters' were hungrier generally and ate more after the set meal. Also, the 'hunters' had a greater preference for fat, and found that carbohydrates were less satisfying than for the 'gatherers'. This study is particularly interesting because it clearly mirrors what is so often found in practice: namely, that 'hunters' tend to be hungry individuals who gravitate to fatty food more than 'gatherers'.

The authors of this study concluded that the distinction between the two groups might arise from physiological differences which may reflect a system adapted to deal with a particular type of diet. They subsequently went on to suggest that, where healthy weight-maintenance is concerned, different people clearly require different strategies.[11]

Put all of this together and there's compelling evidence to show that there is considerable individuality in our biochemistry and metabolisms, and that this influences our nutritional requirements. We have seen that individuals can fall on a spectrum ranging from 'hunters' to 'gatherers'. Those falling near the middle of the spectrum can be classed as 'hunter-gatherers'. In the next chapter we're going to explore further the characteristics of these different types of people.

Have These Differences Got Anything to Do with Blood Group?

In recent times the concept that different diets suit different people has been popularized through an approach based on blood group. There are four main blood groups based on what are known as 'antigens' on the surface of the red blood cells: type A (have 'A' antigens on their cells), type B (have 'B' antigens on their cells), type AB (have both) and type O (have neither). According to Dr Peter D'Adamo, author of the *Eat Right for Your Type* series of books, the foods that are best for us are determined by the antigens on our cells.

His reasoning is based on substances on the surface of foods known as 'lectins'. Basically, lectins have the capacity to react with blood antigens, and this can cause red blood cells to clump together, which can lead to any number of ills including fatigue and chronic disease. According to Dr D'Adamo, the foods we react to are largely determined by the antigens found on our red blood cells. Those of O blood type (which is thought to be the first blood group that came into existence) are best suited to a diet devoid of grain and dairy products. Groups A, B and AB, Dr D'Adamo says, came later and are therefore better adapted, to varying degrees, to these more recent additions to our diet. Dr D'Adamo claims not only that different blood types developed at different points during our evolution, but that the predominant diet at their time of origin reflects the ideal diet for an individual of that blood type.

This may sound a decent enough theory, except there are a few problems with it. First, it simply isn't established *when* different blood groups came about, which casts considerable doubt on the validity of one of the blood group diet's major tenets. Also, if blood groups A, B and AB only came about since we converted from hunter-gathering to farming, then their appearance was very recent in evolutionary terms. Let's not forget, though, that evolution is a very slow process. Genetically, we're more than 99.9 per cent the same as when we introduced farming. In light of these facts, it doesn't seem particularly likely that any of us is particularly well adapted to the diets assigned by Dr D'Adamo to those of blood types A, B and AB.

Another deficiency of this diet relates to the blood types themselves. The ABO group of antigens are just one way to type blood; there are literally dozens of other antigens on the surface of the blood cells. Following Dr D'Adamo's logic, is it not possible that these also developed at different times during our evolution, and therefore influence our dietary requirements? These other antigens are not embraced in Dr D'Adamo's approach.

Another issue with the blood-type approach is that it seems to be based on experiments in which lectins from food have been mixed with blood in the *test tube*. This is important because these experiments do not reflect what happens in nature. Under normal circumstances lectins are not injected into the bloodstream, but are *eaten*. This gives the body an opportunity to inactivate the lectins through the process of digestion. Also, the gut wall may provide some protection by providing a physical barrier against the absorption of lectins into the system. Lectins may also be deactivated even before they get into the gut by the way in which foods are prepared and cooked.

There is no doubt in my mind, however, that food-sensitivity issues do exist. Poor digestion, 'leaky' gut, and the eating of foods to which we are not well adapted are all risk factors for this. For a more thorough explanation of this phenomenon and advice about its diagnosis and management, see Appendix A. However, discerning broad patterns of food sensitivity by mixing lectins with blood *outside* the body is unlikely to bring us answers that reflect reality.

Another potential deficiency of the blood-type approach is that, while it focuses on lectins, there are several other ways in which the body can react to foods. For example, the body's immune cells (known as T-cells) can react to food and produce antibodies of more than one type (the two main types in this regard are known as IgE and IgG antibodies). Such reactions, which are clearly important for assessing food suitability, are just not taken into consideration in the lectin-based 'blood group' approach.

None of this means that taking Dr D'Adamo's advice will not help some people. The most common blood group, 'O', is advised to eat what amounts to a dairy- and grain-free diet. Bearing in mind the very frequent role these foods play in health issues generally (see Chapter 4, Against the Grain and Chapter 6, Slaying the Sacred Cow for more details) then the 'type O' approach is likely to help a lot of people. Also, Dr D'Adamo advises not just the Os but also the As and Bs to eliminate major offenders in the diet such as commercially produced bread, biscuits, pasta and cereals. These foods are generally bad for health for myriad reasons (again, see Chapter 4), and it's therefore no wonder that individuals usually feel better for getting them out of their diet. I wholeheartedly agree with Dr D'Adamo that there is a need for dietary individualization, but the fact is this has little or nothing to do with blood group.

The Bottom Line

- Although we can draw some broad conclusions about what it means to eat a healthy diet, the varying circumstances of our past suggests that our 'ideal' diet varies from individual to individual.

- Anecdotal and scientific evidence shows that there is significant variation in how individuals respond to a given diet.

- Science shows that there is considerable variation in our ability to metabolize food, including fat.

- Scientists have identified two broad types of individual: those who tend to metabolize fat efficiently and are less prone to weight gain ('hunters'), and those who are not efficient metabolizers of fat and are more prone to weight gain ('gatherers').

- 'Hunters' generally have higher heart rates and metabolic rates, and seem to be able to increase their metabolism of fat in response to increased fat intake.

- Compared to 'gatherers', 'hunters' tend to be hungrier and gain more satisfaction from eating fat.

- 'Gatherers' generally have lower heart rates and metabolic rates and do not seem to be able to increase their metabolism of fat in response to increased fat intake.

- Compared to 'hunters', 'gatherers' tend to be less hungry and gain less satisfaction from eating fat.

- Because of variation in our nutritional needs, one man's meat can indeed be another's poison.

Chapter 13 A World of Difference

As we discovered in the last chapter, not only do different diets seem to suit different types of people, but certain characteristics tend to be shared by people of the same type. In this chapter we're going to take a closer look at the typical characteristics of these different types. It is these characteristics that are used as the basis of a questionnaire you can use to determine whether you are a 'hunter', 'gatherer' or 'hunter-gatherer' (see page 144).

'Hunter' Characteristics

General Metabolism
'Hunters' tend to have relatively rapid metabolisms, and are generally efficient converters of food (including fat) into energy.

Body Shape and Size
Because of their brisk metabolisms, 'hunters' can be reasonably resistant to weight gain. In fact, some 'hunters' may even feel 'underweight' and struggle to maintain their weight.

It is possible for 'hunters' to gain weight, especially if a relatively sedentary lifestyle is coupled with a diet that fails to meet their needs. Many 'hunters' who gain weight have done so largely as a result of eating a supposedly 'healthy' diet low in fat and high in carbohydrates.

When 'hunters' gain weight, this typically accumulates around the middle of the body. For this reason, overweight 'hunters' tend to have big waists and high waist-to-hip ratios. More about this type of weight gain – known as 'abdominal obesity' – can be found in Chapter 4 (Against the Grain).

Appetite

'Hunters' tend to burn fuel rapidly, and consequently tend to be hungry individuals who do best eating quite regularly. 'Hunters' usually *like* food and look forward to eating.

When 'hunters' skip meals, the level of blood sugar in the bloodstream can drop, sometimes precipitously. This can cause symptoms of sudden hunger, weakness, shakiness, anxiety and irritability. However, to a degree this can be offset by being busy or stressed, as this will help fuel the body internally through the mobilization of fuel stores (see Chapter 11 for more details about this).

Food Preferences

'Hunters' generally like fat and can even crave it. To a 'hunter', eating fat is a bit like putting a dry log or shovelful of coal on a raging fire. As a result, 'hunters' generally find that fatty foods are sustaining and effective for satis-fying their appetites. They usually like and do well on dark, fatty meats such as beef, lamb, duck, venison and the leg meat of chicken and turkey.

The relatively rapid metabolism of the 'hunter' will tend to burn carbo-hydrates very rapidly. Because of this, 'hunters' tend not to feel satisfied or sustained by carbohydrate-rich foods such as fruits, vegetarian/vegan food or grain-based meals (e.g. pasta, risotto, sandwiches, breakfast cereals). To a 'hunter', eating these foods is akin to putting newspaper or sawdust on a raging fire: they will usually get an immediate boost of energy and some satisfaction of their appetite, but the effects tend to be short-lived.

'Hunters' can find themselves craving sweet foods such as biscuits or chocolate. Unfortunately, once they start eating sweet foods, they can find it difficult to stop.

'Hunters' can also be prone to craving salty foods such as salted peanuts, sausages and salami.

Other Nutritional Characteristics

'Hunters' tend to feel better if they eat between meals, but generally do not do well by eating fruit as a snack. They will usually do better on something fattier such as nuts.

'Hunters' tend to prefer cooked vegetables and feel better after cooked, rather than raw, vegetables. This is particularly the case if the vegetables include added fat in the form of olive oil or butter. Salad is generally less satisfying for 'hunters', and it's common for them to feel hungry quite soon after a salad, even if it contains meat or fish.

Response to Caffeine
'Hunters' don't tend to do well on caffeine. They may find it's relatively easy to overdose on caffeinated coffee and/or tea, and feel 'wired' as a result. 'Hunters' can find caffeine quite addictive, and may also find that it doesn't take too much of it to disrupt their sleep.

Energy
'Hunters' tend to be high-energy individuals, and often like to be 'on the go'. In time, though, 'hunters' can exhaust themselves. This is particularly the case when an inappropriate diet is coupled with factors such as excesses of stress, long working hours and not enough sleep. One specific imbalance that 'hunters' tend to be prone to is weakness in the adrenal glands – the organs that sit on top of the kidneys and are the chief glands in the body responsible for dealing with stress. Features suggestive of adrenal weakness include fatigue, fatigue that is worsened by stress or strenuous exercise, cravings for salt and/or sugar and a tendency towards allergic conditions such as hay fever. (More details about this condition, and how to diagnose and treat it, can be found in Appendix C.)

Sleep Habits
Generally speaking, 'hunters' are able to get by on relatively low amounts of sleep (7 hours or less). In the long term, though, this may contribute to a weakening of the body (see 'Energy' section, above).

Psychological Characteristics
'Hunters' tend to be relatively quick thinkers, may even thrive on the feeling of having a lot to do, and often attempt to do more than one thing at a time. Generally speaking, 'hunters' tend to be 'driven', 'time-urgent' individuals who often endeavour to pack as much as possible (sometimes too much!) into each day.

Mood
The quick mind and generally high-energy characteristics of 'hunters' make them prone to anxiety.

Temperature Preference

'Hunters' tend to be on the warm side, and may feel uncomfortable in hot weather.

Other 'Hunter' Features

Most things go quickly in the 'hunter's' body. Other features characteristic of this type include frequent bowel motions (usually, at least once a day), oily skin, oily hair, good circulation, and relatively rapid pulse rates. Their tendency to have fast metabolisms means that 'hunters' use up oxygen quite quickly, and they generally find it difficult to hold their breath for extended periods.

'Gatherer' Characteristics

General Metabolism

'Gatherers' tend to have relatively slow metabolisms. In general terms, they do not burn food particularly quickly in the body, and can therefore be prone to weight gain. Some find it difficult to lose weight, too.

Body Shape and Size

Not all 'gatherers' are overweight. However, when excess weight is present, this tends to be distributed throughout the body.

Appetite

'Gatherers' are often not very hungry, and can often go quite long periods of time without eating. They often find no 'need' to eat between meals.

Food Preferences

'Gatherers' tend to be drawn to foods relatively low in fat, including fruits, vegetables, beans and lentils. To a 'gatherer', eating these plant-based foods is a bit like putting small pieces of wood on a gently burning fire. These foods will tend to energize 'gatherers' more than heavier, fattier foods, which can tend to overwhelm their internal 'fire'.

Other Nutritional Characteristics

'Gatherers' tend not to need to eat between meals, but if they do they will often find fresh fruit will satisfy them.

'Gatherers' do well on a vegetable-rich diet, including raw vegetables such as salad. They tend not to feel as well on cooked vegetables with added fat such as olive oil or butter.

Response to Caffeine
'Gatherers' tend to do quite well on caffeine. They don't tend to get much of a 'kick' from drinking coffee or tea, tend not to find these drinks addictive, and often are able to consume a fair amount of caffeine without it disrupting their sleep.

Energy
'Gatherers' tend not to be particularly 'high energy' people, though they often have very good stamina. 'Gatherers' may not be particularly fast, but they can often keep going throughout the day.

One specific imbalance that 'gatherers' tend to be prone to is weakness in the thyroid gland – the organ chiefly responsible for regulating the body's metabolism. Features suggestive of this include the inability to lose weight, sensitivity to cold, cold hands and/or feet, dry skin, dry hair, a tendency to constipation, and low mood. (More details about this condition, and how to diagnose and treat it, can be found in Appendix D.)

Sleep Habits
'Gatherers' tend to need relatively long periods of sleep – often 8 hours or more a night are necessary for these individuals to feel properly rested.

Psychological Characteristics
'Gatherers' generally prefer to move methodically from one job or activity to the next, and tend not to attempt to do too many things at once. Generally speaking, 'gatherers' take a relatively laid-back attitude to life.

Mood
'Gatherers' tend to be prone to low mood and depression.

Temperature Preference
'Gatherers' tend to be on the cold side, and usually prefer warm weather.

Other 'Gatherer' Features

Most things go relatively slowly in the 'gatherer's' body. Other features characteristic of this type include a tendency to infrequent bowel motions (often, less than once a day), dry skin, dry hair, poor circulation, and relatively slow pulse rates. Their tendency to have slow metabolisms means that 'gatherers' use up oxygen quite slowly, and they generally find it easier than 'hunters' to hold their breath for extended periods.

'Hunter-Gatherer' Characteristics

The characteristics of the typical 'hunter-gatherer' fall in between those of the 'hunters' and 'gatherers'.

The Bottom Line

- The characteristics of individuals and their ideal diets can be broadly divided into three categories: 'hunters', 'gatherers', and 'hunter-gatherers'.

- Generally, 'hunters' tend to have relatively brisk metabolisms, are hungry individuals, and have rapid pulse rates and a tendency to put on weight around the middle of the body.

- Generally, 'gatherers' tend to have relatively slow metabolisms, are not very hungry individuals and have slow pulse rates and a tendency to accumulate weight all over their body.

- The characteristics of the 'hunter-gatherer' fall in between those of the 'hunters' and 'gatherers'.

Chapter 14 **Take the Test**

In the preceding two chapters we have explored the scientific basis for the idea of dietary individualization, as well as some of the common characteristics of different types of individuals. Now, we're going to use this information to discover what type *you* are.

The characteristics that set 'hunters', 'gatherers', and 'hunter-gatherers' apart have been used to construct this questionnaire. There are 30 questions, each of which has five potential answers: 1–5. Most questions only have answers written against numbers 1, 3 and 5. If one of these answers seems to describe you quite accurately, mark the box next to this answer. Sometimes, you may feel that the answer that best reflects you is somewhere in between 1 and 3, in which case mark this as '2'. Similarly, if you feel the most accurate answer for you falls between 3 and 5, mark '4'. You may occasionally feel you do not know what answer to give. It is important that you do not leave these questions, but mark your answer as '3'.

While this questionnaire is designed to be as user-friendly as possible, it is important that you assign some quiet time to answer it. You'll almost certainly get a more accurate result if you are not feeling time-pressured or preoccupied when you complete the questionnaire.

Once you have answered all the questions, simply add up the numbers that correspond to the answers you have given – answers 1, 2, 3, 4 and 5 gain 1, 2, 3, 4 and 5 points respectively. Total scores will vary between 30 and 150.

Questionnaire

1. How often do you usually eat each day?

1. Once or twice including snacks ☑
2. ☐
3. Three meals a day with generally no snacks ☐
4. ☐
5. Three meals a day with usually one or two snacks in between ☐

2. If you were to get peckish between meals, what effect would drinking a glass of fruit juice or eating a piece of fruit generally have on you?

1. It would energize you, satisfy your appetite, and get you comfortably through to the next meal ☑
2. ☐
3. It would sustain you reasonably well but might be better supplemented with a 'heavier' food such as nuts/don't know ☐
4. ☐
5. It would not really satisfy you at all, and possibly leave you feeling even hungrier ☐

3. What effect is eating a relatively 'light' lunch such as chicken or tuna salad or a vegetarian dish likely to have on you?

1. You would be well energized throughout the afternoon and unlikely to be in need of food until dinner ☐
2. ☐
3. You would be reasonably well energized but likely to need a snack before dinner/don't know ☑
4. ☐
5. You would be hungry by the end of the afternoon, and almost definitely in need of a snack before dinner ☐

4. What sort of breakfast seems to energize you for the morning and is most likely to get you to lunch without the need to eat again?

1. Little or no breakfast or one based on fruit, cereal and/or toast ☑
2. ☐
3. A mix of fat-rich and lighter foods such as eggs and toast/don't know ☐

4.   ☐

5. A 'hearty' breakfast comprising fatty foods such as bacon, sausage and
   egg   ☐

5. If you were going out for a celebratory meal, and felt unrestricted by any nutritional or health concerns, what sort of meal would you tend to choose?

1. Relatively light foods such as vegetarian dishes, with plenty of
   vegetables and/or grains (such as rice or pasta) but little in the
   way of meat or oily fish   ☐

2.   ☐

3. Dishes containing chicken or fish/don't know   ☑

4.   ☐

5. Dishes containing dark meat such as beef (e.g. steak), lamb or
   duck   ☐

6. What is your appetite for salt (ignoring any health advice you may be aware of regarding salt)?

1. You don't like salty foods and rarely, if ever, add it to food   ☑

2.   ☐

3. You don't care much for salt one way or the other/don't know   ☐

4.   ☐

5. You tend to enjoy salty foods, and quite often add salt to food
   during cooking or at the table   ☐

7. What's your general attitude to food and eating?

1. You're not that interested in food, and eating is not something
   you're particularly focused on   ☐

2.   ☐

3. You enjoy food, but it's not something you are particularly
   focused on/don't know   ☐

4.   ☐

5. You enjoy food a lot, like eating, and tend to look forward to
   meals   ☐

8. How hungry do you tend to be at breakfast?

1. Not at all hungry   ☐

2. ☐

3. Moderately hungry/don't know ☑3

4. ☐

5. Very hungry/ravenous ☐

9. How hungry do you tend to be at lunch?

1. Not at all hungry ☐

2. ☐

3. Moderately hungry/don't know ☑3

4. ☐

5. Very hungry/ravenous ☐

10. How hungry do you tend to be at dinner?

1. Not at all hungry ☐

2. ☐

3. Moderately hungry/don't know ☑3

4. ☐

5. Very hungry/ravenous ☐

11. What sort of portion sizes tend to satisfy you?

1. You are generally satisfied with small portions, and rarely have second helpings ☐

2. ☐

3. You are generally satisfied with moderate portions, and tend not to have second helpings/don't know ☑3

4. ☐

5. You like a full plate, feel the need to eat plenty to satisfy your appetite and are often inclined to have second helpings if they're on offer ☐

12. What effect does eating a relatively large evening meal tend to have on your sleep?

1. Tends to disturb your sleep ☐

2. ☐

3. Has no particular effect on your sleep/don't know ☑3

4. ☐

5. Tends to improve your sleep ☐

13. If a whole chicken or turkey was on offer at a meal, would you prefer...?

   1. The breast (lighter) meat (also answer '1' if you are vegetarian) ☐

   2. ☐

   3. Not bothered either way/don't know ☐

   4. ☐

   5. The leg (darker) meat ☑5

14. Which of these foods do you feel enhance your well-being and energy?

   1. Relatively low-fat foods such as fruits, vegetables and grain (such as bread, rice and pasta) ☐

   2. ☐

   3. A mix of foods such as meat, fish, vegetables and grain (such as bread, rice and pasta)/don't know ☑

   4. ☐

   5. Heavy foods such as meat, particularly red meats such as beef, lamb or duck ☐

15. Which of these foods tend to enhance your mental energy and focus?

   1. Relatively low-fat foods such as fruit, vegetables and grain (such as bread, rice and pasta) ☐

   2. ☐

   3. A mix of foods such as meat, fish, vegetables and grain (such as bread, rice and pasta)/don't know ☑

   4. ☐

   5. Heavy foods such as meat, particularly red meats such as beef, lamb or duck ☐

16. What effect does eating very sweet foods such as chocolate or biscuits have on your subsequent appetite for these foods?

   1. You can eat a relatively small amount of such foods without feeling a need for more ☐

   2. ☐

   3. Once you start, you may find it difficult to stop eating these sorts of foods/don't know ☑

   4. ☐

   5. Once you start, you often find it difficult to stop eating these sorts of foods and can find yourself 'gorging' on them ☐

17. What effect does drinking caffeinated coffee have on you?

1. You feel generally well on coffee and, as long as you don't overdo it, tend not to feel either 'wired' or jittery ☑

2. ☐

3. You feel generally well on coffee, as long as you do not drink more than 2–4 cups a day/don't know ☐

4. ☐

5. You quite easily find yourself feeling 'wired' or jittery if you drink caffeinated coffee ☐

18. How do you feel if lunch, for some reason, is delayed by a couple of hours?

1. You might be hungry, but otherwise you would feel fine ☑

2. ☐

3. You would tend to get hungry and are also likely to feel like your energy levels and/or mood are affected adversely/don't know ☐

4. ☐

5. You would tend to get very hungry and might also feel quite weak, shaky or irritable ☐

19. Which of these represents your favourite dessert/pudding (ignoring any health concerns you may be aware of)?

1. Sweet-tasting and/or fruit-based puddings such as fruit, fruit tart, apple crumble, cake or gateaux ☑

2. ☐

3. No particular favourite dessert/don't know ☐

4. ☐

5. Cheesecake or cheese ☐

20. What's your attitude to butter and buttery sauces (ignoring any health concerns you may have about these foods)?

1. You don't like butter and tend to find buttery sauces too rich for your taste ☐

2. ☐

3. You can take or leave butter or buttery sauces/don't know ☑

4. ☐

5. You like butter and/or buttery sauces ☐

21. Do you tend to wake in the night?

1. You very rarely or never wake in the night unless disturbed or need to go to the toilet ☐
2. ☐
3. You can occasionally find yourself awake in the middle of the night for no obvious reason/don't know ☑
4. ☐
5. You can often find yourself wake at about 3.00 or 4.00 a.m., and sometimes have difficulty getting back to sleep again ☐

22. How would you describe your wound-healing potential?

1. Your wound healing tends to be on the slow side ☐
2. ☐
3. Your wound-healing potential does not seem to be either slower or quicker than others/don't know ☑
4. ☐
5. Your wound healing tends to be rapid ☐

23. On average, how often do you open your bowels?

1. Less than once a day ☑
2. ☐
3. Once a day/don't know ☐
4. ☐
5. More than once a day ☐

24. How would you describe the condition of your skin and hair?

1. Generally dry ☑
2. ☐
3. Neither dry nor oily/don't know ☐
4. ☐
5. Generally oily ☐

25. How would you describe your circulation?

1. You tend to suffer from cold hands and/or feet ☑
2. ☐
3. Your hands and feet do not tend to be particularly warm or cold/ don't know ☐

4. □

5. You tend to have warm hands and/or feet □

26. How would you describe your personality?
1. You do not feel particularly 'driven' or 'time-urgent', and believe you take a relatively laid-back attitude to life □

2. □

3. You do not feel either particularly 'driven' or laid-back/don't know □

4. □

5. You feel quite 'driven' or 'time-urgent', and generally attempt to get the most out of each day ⑤

27. What sort of weather do you prefer?
1. You definitely prefer warm weather over cold ①

2. □

3. You have no preference/don't know □

4. □

5. You definitely prefer cold weather over warm □

28. In the rested state, what is your pulse rate in beats per minute? (see instructions on page 152 on how to measure your pulse rate)
1. less than 60 □

2. 60–64 □

3. 65–70 □

4. 71–75 □

5. 76 or more ⑤

29. After taking a few deep breaths, how long can you comfortably hold your breath for?
1. 60 or more seconds □

2. 50–59 seconds □

3. 40–49 seconds □

4. 30–39 seconds ④

5. fewer than 30 seconds □

30. For men only: What is your waist-to-hip ratio? (see instructions on page 152 for how to measure your waist-to-hip ratio)

1. less than 0.89 ☐
2. 0.89–0.92 ☐
3. 0.93–0.95 ☐
4. 0.96–0.99 ☐
5. more than 0.99 ☐

30. For women only: What is your waist-to-hip ratio? (see instructions on page 152 for how to measure your waist-to-hip ratio)

1. less than 0.80 ☐
2. 0.80–0.83 ☑
3. 0.84–0.86 ☐
4. 0.87–0.90 ☐
5. more than 0.90 ☐

Score Interpretation

30–75   'Gatherer' ☐
76–105   'Hunter-gatherer' ☑
106–150 'Hunter' ☐

A Word about Interpreting Your Test Score

This questionnaire is designed to help determine which of the three types ('hunter', 'gatherer', 'hunter-gatherer') you are. These types are obviously part of a spectrum. What this means is that if it turns out your score is 78, then while this marks you out as a 'hunter-gatherer', there's probably more 'gatherer' in you, than 'hunter'. By the same token, a score of 103 suggests more 'hunter' than 'gatherer'. In addition to determining your type, keeping in mind where you fall on the spectrum can help you fine-tune your diet in a way that best meets your nutritional needs.

How to Take Your Pulse

The artery that is easiest to use for taking your pulse is the radial artery which is located on the palm side of your wrist in line with your thumb. To take your pulse, place the index and middle finger of your other hand gently on this artery. Count the beats for 30 seconds; then double the result to get the number of beats per minute.

How to Measure Your Waist-to-hip Ratio

Measure the circumference (in either cm or inches) of your waist at the level of your naval or just above. Measure the circumference around your buttocks at their widest point in the same units. Divide the first measurement by the second.

Chapter 15 **What Is There To Eat?**

Now that you know whether you are a 'hunter', 'hunter-gatherer' or 'gatherer', we can go on to look at the sorts of foods and meals that are going to best suit your needs. This chapter starts with some broad dietary recommendations for each type. Tables that summarize this advice are provided for easy reference. After this, suggestions are given for breakfast, lunch and dinner for each type. Finally, recipes designed specifically for each type can be found starting on page 179.

The 'Hunter' Diet

Meat and Fish

'Hunters' tend to do well on relatively fatty, protein-rich foods. Good foods to emphasize in the diet therefore include beef, lamb, duck, chicken-leg meat and quality sausages or burgers (preferably homemade). Fish, ideally, should be oily (e.g. salmon, trout, mackerel, sardines). Seafood is a good choice, too.

'Hunters' will generally not do quite as well on 'lean' meats such as chicken and turkey breast or non-oily and white fish such as cod, plaice and haddock. These, however, can be eaten in moderation, as long as they are balanced by other, fattier, 'heavier' meat and fish eaten elsewhere in the diet.

Fruits and Vegetables

As far as vegetables go, 'hunters' will generally benefit most from highly nutritious, relatively low-GI varieties that grow above the ground such as broccoli, green beans, spinach and asparagus. Root vegetables such as potatoes, carrots, parsnips and turnips can be eaten, though these should

Table 15.1 'Hunter' Dietary Recommendations

Meat	Fish and seafood	Vegetables	Fruit
Foods to emphasize in the diet			
Beef	*Oily fish such as:*	Vegetables growing	Olives
Lamb	Salmon	above the ground	Avocados
Venison	Trout	such as:	
Duck	Mackerel	Broccoli	
Chicken and turkey	Herring	Cabbage	
leg meat	Sardines	Cauliflower	
Liver	Anchovy	French beans	
Quality and	*Shellfish such as:*	Mange tout	
homemade	Mussels	Roast/cooked	
sausages and	Crab	tomatoes	
burgers	Lobster	Courgette	
	Crayfish	Spinach	
	Prawns	Kale	
		Asparagus	
Foods to eat in moderation			
Less fatty cuts such	Non 'oily' fish such	*Root vegetables such as:*	Apples
as:	as:	Potatoes	Pears
Chicken and turkey	Swordfish	Carrots	Citrus fruits
breast	Tuna	Parsnip	Berries
Lean beef	Cod	Swede	Bananas
Lean pork	Plaice	Turnips	Mangoes
	Sole	*Raw and salad*	Grapes
	Haddock	*vegetables such as:*	Pineapple
	Halibut	Lettuce	Dried fruit
		Tomato	
		Celery	
		Cucumber	
		Shredded carrot	
Foods to avoid			

'Hunter' Dietary Recommendations

Dairy products other than butter	Grains	Oils, fats and spreads	Other foods	Beverages
		Butter Extra-virgin olive oil	Nuts and seeds of all forms, preferably raw (unroasted)	Water Herbal tea
Goat's and sheep's milk, yoghurt and cheese	*Unrefined* *relatively low GI* *grains, such as:* Oats Rye (e.g. whole rye bread) Brown rice		Eggs Beans and lentils	Coffee and tea
Cow's milk, yoghurt and cheese	High-GI and -GL grains such as wheat, corn and white rice	Margarine		Fruit juice and smoothies Alcoholic beverages

be seen as a minor accompaniment to a meal. Salad vegetables can be eaten, though most 'hunters' will not feel as sustained on these as on cooked vegetables, especially those with added olive oil or butter.

'Hunters' do not tend to do well on fruit, but may have some in the form of low-GI fruits such as apples, pears and berries. Dried fruit and higher-GI fruits such as bananas, mangoes and pineapples can be eaten, too, but in limited quantities. Avocados and olives, on account of their high fat and protein content, are good forms of fruit for 'hunters'.

Dairy Products

'Hunters' tend to tolerate dairy products quite well, especially butter and full-fat yoghurt. 'Hunters' will generally tolerate goat's and sheep's products better than cow's products. These foods can be included in the diet in moderation.

Grains

'Hunters' do not do well on grains, but will usually tolerate some of these in the form of oats, rye (e.g. whole rye bread) and brown rice. 'Hunters' should avoid, as much as possible, high-GI/GL grains such as wheat (which they are often sensitive to as well), corn and white rice.

Oils, Fats and Spreads

Butter and extra-virgin olive oil can be used quite liberally in the diet, but margarine (of all types) should be avoided.

Beans and Lentils

Moderate amounts of beans and lentils are an alternative to grains for 'hunters'. Generally speaking, these are much better eaten as an accompaniment to food or as a meal ingredient (e.g. beans or lentils in soups or stews) rather than as the main ingredient in a recipe or meal.

Other Foods

Nuts and seeds can be emphasized in the 'hunter' diet. In particular, these represent a good snack choice for this type. Ideally, nuts and seeds should be had in their raw (unroasted) form. The roasting of nuts can damage the fats they contain and will tend to reduce their nutritional value. Eggs may be eaten in moderation, too.

Beverages

Good drinks for 'hunters' include water and herbal tea.

'Hunters' will generally tolerate coffee and tea to some extent. This will depend on an individual's ability to metabolize caffeine, but most 'hunters' will be able to tolerate 1–3 cups of coffee or tea a day, as long as these are not drunk later than lunchtime.

Drinks for 'hunters' to avoid include fruit juices, smoothies and alcoholic drinks. Of the alcoholic drinks, those with the lowest GI/GL are best. Examples include whiskey and soda, and vodka, lime and soda.

The 'Hunter-Gatherer' Diet

Meat and Fish

'Hunter-gatherers' will generally do well on a mix of meats, fish and seafood, including fattier and lower-fat varieties. Suitable foods include beef, chicken, turkey, pork, lamb, and oily and white fish.

Fruits and Vegetables

'Hunter-gatherers' will tend to do well on all forms of vegetables, including root vegetables such as potatoes and parsnips. In general, the emphasis should be on vegetables that grow above the ground such as broccoli, cabbage, French beans and salad vegetables. A mix of cooked and raw vegetables tends to suit 'hunter-gatherers' well.

'Hunter-gatherers' tend to do best on relatively low-GI/GL fruits such as apples, pears and berries. Olives and avocados can also be eaten. Dried fruit and relatively high-GI fruit such as bananas, pineapples and grapes can be eaten in moderation.

Dairy Products

'Hunter-gatherers' tend to tolerate dairy products reasonably well. Goat's and sheep's products, particularly yoghurt, are usually tolerated better than cow's products. These foods can be included in the diet in moderation.

Grains

'Hunter-gatherers' tolerate grains reasonably well, but these are best had in the form of oats, rye (e.g. whole rye bread) and brown rice. 'Hunter-gatherers'

Table 15.2 'Hunter-Gatherer' Dietary Recommendations

Meat	Fish and seafood	Vegetables	Fruit
Foods to emphasize in the diet			
A mix of all forms	A mix of all forms	A mix of all forms including cooked and raw	Low-glycaemic index fruits such as: Apples Pears Citrus fruits Berries Olives Avocado
Foods to eat in moderation			
			Higher-GI and -GL fruits such as: Bananas Mangoes Grapes Pineapples Dried fruit
Foods to avoid			

'Hunter-Gatherer' Dietary Recommendations

Dairy products other than butter	Grains	Oils, fats and spreads	Other foods	Beverages
		Extra-virgin olive oil		Water Herbal tea
Goat's and sheep's milk, yoghurt and cheese	Unrefined, relatively low-GI grains such as: Oats Whole rye bread Brown rice	Butter	Nuts and seeds of all forms, preferably raw (unroasted) Eggs Beans and lentils	Coffee and tea Fruit smoothies
Cow's milk, yoghurt and cheese	High-GI and -GL grains such as wheat, corn and white rice	Margarine		Fruit juice Alcoholic beverages

should avoid high-GI/GL grains such as wheat (which they are often sensitive to as well), corn and white rice.

Oils, Fats and Spreads
Extra-virgin olive oil can be used liberally in the diet, and butter can be used in moderation. Margarine (of all types) should be avoided.

Other Foods
Nuts and seeds can be eaten in moderation, though, ideally, these should be eaten in their raw (unroasted) form. The roasting of nuts can damage the fats they contain and will tend to reduce their nutritional value.

Eggs can also be eaten in moderation by 'hunter-gatherers'.

Beans and Lentils
Moderate amounts of beans and lentils are an alternative to grains for 'hunter-gatherers'. Generally speaking, these are better had as an accompaniment to food or as a meal ingredient (e.g. beans or lentils as part of a heartier soup or stew) rather than as the main ingredient in a recipe or meal.

Beverages
Good drinks for 'hunter-gatherers' include water and herbal tea.

'Hunter-gatherers' will generally tolerate coffee and tea quite well. This will depend on an individual's ability to metabolize caffeine, but most 'hunter-gatherers' are able to tolerate 2–4 cups of coffee or tea a day, as long as it is not drunk too late in the day.

Smoothies, based on whole fruit, can be drunk in moderation.

Drinks for 'hunter-gatherers' to avoid include fruit juice and alcoholic drinks. Of the alcoholic drinks, those with the lowest GI/GL are best. Examples include whiskey and soda and vodka, lime and soda.

The 'Gatherer' Diet

Meat and Fish
'Gatherers' tend to do well on a relatively light diet, and will usually do best on moderate amounts of lean meats, fish (including some oily fish) and seafood. Heavier, fattier meats such as sausages, lamb and game meats should be avoided.

Fruits and Vegetables

'Gatherers' should emphasize fruit and vegetables in the diet in all forms.

Generally, 'gatherers' will feel better when consuming raw rather than cooked vegetables.

Olives and avocados, on account of their fatty nature, should be consumed only in moderation.

Dairy Products

'Gatherers' tend to be sensitive to dairy products, especially those based on cow's milk. Goat's products, particularly yoghurt, are usually tolerated better. These foods can be included in the diet in moderation.

Grains

'Gatherers' tolerate grains reasonably well, but these should be in the form of relatively low-GI foods that are unlikely to trigger food-sensitivity reactions – such as oats, rye (e.g. whole rye bread) and brown rice. 'Gatherers' should generally avoid high-GI/GL grains such as wheat (which they can be sensitive to as well), corn and white rice.

Oils, Fats and Spreads

Extra-virgin olive oil can be consumed in moderation and butter can be used sparingly in the diet. Margarine (of all types) should be avoided.

Other Foods

Nuts and seeds can be eaten in moderation by 'gatherers', though, ideally, these should be eaten in their raw (unroasted) form. The roasting of nuts can damage the fats they contain and will tend to reduce their nutritional value.

Eggs can also be eaten in moderation by 'gatherers'.

Beans and Lentils

Beans and lentils are generally good foods for 'gatherers', and can form the basis/main ingredient for a meal (e.g. lentil soup or bean stew).

Beverages

Good drinks for 'gatherers' include water and herbal tea.

Table 15.3 'Gatherer' Dietary Recommendations

Meat	Fish and seafood	Vegetables	Fruit
Foods to emphasize in the diet			
		A mix of all types including cooked and raw	A mix of all types
Foods to eat in moderation			
Light and less fatty cuts such as: Chicken and turkey breast	A mix of all types of fish and seafood		Olives Avocado
Foods to avoid			
Beef Lamb Venison Chicken and turkey leg meat Liver Quality and homemade sausages and burgers			

'Gatherer' Dietary Recommendations

Dairy products other than butter	Grains	Oils, fats and spreads	Other foods	Beverages
			Beans and lentils	Water Herbal tea
Goat's and sheep's milk, yoghurt and cheese	Unrefined, relatively low-GI grains such as: Oats Rye (e.g. whole rye bread) Brown rice	Extra-virgin olive oil Butter (may be used sparingly)	Eggs Nuts and seeds, preferably raw (unroasted)	Fruit juices and smoothies Coffee and tea
Cow's milk, yoghurt and cheese	High-GI and -GL grains such as wheat, corn and white rice	Margarine		Alcoholic beverages

'Gatherers' will generally tolerate coffee and tea quite well. This will depend on an individual's ability to metabolize caffeine, but most 'gatherers' are able to tolerate 3–5 cups of coffee or tea a day, as long as they are not drunk too late in the day.

Drinks for 'gatherers' to avoid include fruit juices and alcoholic drinks. Of the alcoholic drinks, those with the lowest GI/GL are best. Examples include whiskey and soda and vodka, lime and soda.

Putting It into Practice

Now that we have an idea of the preferred (and not-so-preferred) foods for each type, we can look at how these recommendations can be put into practice in real life.

A Word about Breakfast

Of all the main meals, I reckon breakfast poses more problems than any other. For a variety of reasons, usual breakfast fare such as toast and/or packet breakfast cereals with milk are not a good choice for any of the types. Neither, of course, are 'breakfast' bars or muffins.

With this in mind, I have put together three variations of what is known as 'Bircher' muesli – named after the Swiss man who invented it. The main ingredients in this dish are plain oats, plain yoghurt (preferably goat's or sheep's), ground nuts and dried fruits.

By varying the relative amounts of ground nuts and dried fruits, the recipe can be adjusted according to your type.

Table 15.4

	'Hunter'		'Hunter-Gatherer'		'Gatherer'	
	Cups	Grams	Cups	Grams	Cups	Grams
Rolled oats	3	300	3	300	3	300
Ground nuts	3	300	2	200	1	100
Dried fruit	1	150	2	300	3	450
Plain yoghurt	2	500	2	500	2	500

The ingredients should be placed in a bowl and mixed with enough water to produce something like the consistency of porridge. This should be put in an airtight container and put in the fridge overnight.

Leaving this muesli overnight helps soften its ingredients, including the nuts and oats, making them more digestible. The live bacteria in the yoghurt will also help to ferment the food slightly, which also enhances its digestibility.

I think this muesli is a very good option for breakfast for a number of reasons. First of all, it is based on a variety of foods that offer a broad range of nutrients. The blend of foods is designed to give a relatively slow release of sugar into the bloodstream. The foods on which this breakfast is based also tend to be some of the best-tolerated foods from a food-intolerance perspective.

One further thing I like about this muesli is that it is *convenient*. The quantities I have specified in the Table are usually enough to last for several days. This muesli generally keeps very well in the fridge, which means that only one or two batches need to be made each week. Once you have the ingredients to hand, each batch takes no more than 5 minutes to put together.

There is quite a lot of room to manoeuvre with regard to the ingredients here if you are keen on variety. For example, there are lots of different types of nuts and/or dried fruits that might be used. Fresh fruit is also an option. Some individuals like, for instance, to add grated apple to the mix. Others might like to add some fresh fruit on top (berries go particularly well).

For those who are sensitive to yoghurt (even goat's yoghurt) I recommend substituting this with either rice milk (for 'gatherers') or nut (e.g. almond) or coconut milk (for 'hunters'). 'Hunter-gatherers' can have either.

Those sensitive to nuts can substitute seeds (e.g. sunflower, pumpkin, sesame) if these are tolerated. Those sensitive to oats may like to try cooked brown rice (this works better than you may imagine), millet flakes or quinoa.

I have suggested other options for breakfast for the different types in the Meal Plans, below, but my advice is to use this muesli as your 'default' breakfast. My experience in practice is that it often really helps to sustain individuals through the morning. More than that, though, I have found that when individuals eat a decent breakfast of this sort, they will usually find that it helps keep their appetite from running out of control later in the day. Not surprisingly, individuals find that this makes eating in accordance with their type so much easier!

Meal Plans

Here are some quick and easy suggestions for breakfast and lunch for the three types. See the Recipes chapter for information on starters and main courses for 'hunters', 'hunter-gatherers', and 'gatherers'.

'Hunters'

Breakfast

Bircher muesli
My recommendation for a good breakfast to be eaten either at home or to take into work and eat on the commute or once at the office.

Poached eggs and smoked salmon (or organic bacon) with tomatoes and mushrooms
I see these options as suggestions for the weekend, where you might be eating slightly later (and be hungrier as a result), and where breakfast/ brunch can be more of an event.

Lunch

Beef or prawn, avocado and salad sandwich(es) made with thinly sliced whole rye bread
Because sandwiches are bread-based I generally don't recommend them, particularly where 'hunters' are concerned. They are, however, very convenient, particularly for those short on time. The trick here is to de-emphasize the bread by using thinly sliced rye bread, and by 'over-filling' the sandwich. Rye bread has a generally lower GI than wheat-based bread. Plus, rye is generally better tolerated (from a food-sensitivity perspective) than wheat.

Chargrilled beef or lamb steak with buttered, steamed green vegetables
This meal may look like hard work, but with a griddle pan and steamer you should be able to rustle it up in 10–15 minutes.

Beef broth and a piece of fruit
A hearty, meat-based soup can be made in bulk and eaten for lunch for two or three days on the trot.

Evening Meal

Steak or lamb chops with cooked vegetables
Like the lunch, this very 'hunter'-ish meal doesn't need to take more than 15 minutes to put together.

Beef or lamb stew and green vegetables
Even quicker would be to prepare a stew or casserole in advance, and just reheat to be served with a green vegetable accompaniment. My suggestion

would be to have a stock of some frozen peas, because these will generally make a very good accompaniment to this sort of dish if you're out of fresh vegetables.

Peppered smoked mackerel or smoked trout with tomato, onion and avocado salad
'Hunters' generally do best on cooked vegetables, but that doesn't mean salad is banned. Here's a good example of a very 'hunter'-ish meal that takes no cooking at all. All it requires is a bit of preparation and perhaps making a dressing based, say, on olive oil and lemon juice. This would, of course, make a very good lunch.

'Hunter-Gatherers'

Breakfast
Bircher muesli
My recommendation for a good breakfast to be eaten either at home or taken into work and eaten on the commute or once at the office.

Poached eggs and smoked salmon (or organic bacon) with tomatoes and a slice of whole rye bread
I see these options as suggestions for the weekend, where you might be eating slightly later (and be hungrier as a result), and where breakfast/ brunch can be more of an event.

Lunch
Salmon, chicken or egg salad sandwich(es) made with thinly sliced whole rye bread
Because sandwiches are bread-based I generally don't recommend them. They are, however, very convenient, particularly for those short on time. The trick here is to de-emphasize the bread by using thinly sliced rye bread, and by over-filling the sandwich. Rye bread has a generally lower GI than wheat-based bread. Plus, rye is generally better tolerated (from a food-sensitivity perspective) than wheat.

Fish or chicken with buttered, steamed green vegetables
This meal may look like hard work, but with a griddle pan and steamer you should be able to rustle it up in 10–15 minutes.

Chicken or turkey broth and a piece of fruit
A meat-based soup can be made in bulk and eaten for lunch for two or three days on the trot.

Evening Meal
Chicken or fish with cooked vegetables and/or salad
Like the lunch, this needn't take more than 15 minutes to put together.

Chicken stew and green vegetables
Even quicker would be to prepare a stew or casserole in advance, and just reheat with some vegetable accompaniment. My suggestion would be to have a stock of some frozen peas, because these will generally make a very good accompaniment to this sort of dish if you're out of fresh vegetables.

Salmon Niçoise
Lettuce, cooked new potatoes, fish, green beans, and olives – an ideal combination of foods for a 'hunter-gatherer'. A recipe for this dish can be found on page 201.

'Gatherers'

Breakfast
Bircher muesli
My recommendation for a good breakfast, to be eaten either at home or perhaps taken into work and eaten on the commute or once at the office.

Plain goat's or sheep's yoghurt with some fresh fruit
For 'gatherers' who are really not very hungry, this represents a perfectly adequate breakfast.

Poached eggs with tomatoes and a slice of whole rye bread
I see this option as something for the weekend, when you might be eating slightly later (and be hungrier as a result) and where breakfast/brunch can be more of an event.

Lunch

Chicken, prawn or egg sandwich(es) made with thinly sliced whole rye bread
While 'gatherers' tend to tolerate grains quite well, I don't recommend that they form the basis of a meal. So, the trick with a sandwich is to de-emphasize the bread by using thinly sliced rye bread, and by over-filling the sandwich. Rye bread has a generally lower GI than wheat-based bread. Plus, rye is generally better tolerated (from a food-sensitivity perspective) than wheat.

Prawn, chicken breast or salmon salad
Light, nutritious and quick to prepare.

Vegetable soup and a piece of fruit
Another quick, light and nutritious lunch for the 'gatherer'.

Evening Meal

Grilled fish or chicken with cooked vegetables and/or salad
A good option for 'gatherers' who eat meat and/or fish.

Winter crumble (the recipe for this can be found on page 218)
A highly nutritious vegan dish that can be prepared in advance and reheated.

Stir-fried vegetables (with prawns or chicken) and brown rice
Another rapid-fire evening meal that is ideal for a 'gatherer'.

Chapter 16 **Looking to the Future**

The True You Diet is based on evolutionary theory, science and, most importantly of all, what works in practice. Working with individuals in the clinical setting has allowed me the privilege of seeing for myself in the real world what is generally effective for attaining optimal health, appropriate weight and vibrant well-being, as well as what isn't.

I see my approach as a doctor as primarily educational. The aim is generally to give my clients, in as few a number of consultations as possible, the advice and support they need to achieve their health goals – not just now, but for the rest of their lives.

However, working with individuals in practice is not always a bowl of cherries. I have seen countless individuals who, at the initial consultation, tell tales of woe about the number of diets they've started and stopped. Each time, any weight they lost has slowly but surely returned, often with a bit of added 'interest' for good measure. Sometimes, I see individuals who seem unable to shift their excess weight no matter what. Incidentally, I usually find that in such individuals the thyroid is at fault (see Appendix D for more details about this).

Also, from time to time, I see former clients who may have done very well for a year or more, who have fallen off the horse and come back to my practice for a 'refresher'. While I'm happy to see a previous patient, I'd be happier if they had fulfilled their health objectives in a way that meant they didn't feel the need to return at all.

Some of this may resonate with you, of course. As I touched on in the Introduction, you may feel as though you have had your fair share of diet success and failure. And if that is indeed the case, then you are clearly not alone. The plethora of diets available out there, and the fact that our collective weight continues to rise rapidly, suggest quite strongly that 'diets' don't work. In fact, there's abundant evidence that, overall, they are a crashing failure.

Because my aim is for *The True You Diet* to be a final destination for you in your quest for healthy eating, a weight you're comfortable with and optimal vitality, I think it's important to look at some of the major reasons why diets don't work out. My aim in this chapter is to offer suggestions, tips and advice designed to help you incorporate the principles of *The True You Diet* permanently into your life. This book may be very much about looking at our nutritional past, but long-term success depends on us keeping an eye on the future, too.

Diet Is a Four-letter Word

This book may have the word 'diet' in the title, but I'm well aware of that word's tarnished reputation. The ineffectiveness of diets has tainted the word. Also, for some, the word 'diet' conjures up images of some strict and unsustainable regime. For this reason I encourage you to interpret the word 'diet' in the title of this book not as something stringent and restrictive that will inevitably come to an end in a few weeks or months, but as a healthy way of eating to be used for your lifelong benefit.

At the same time, I know that most of us don't like the thought of committing to a regime until we know it's something we're actually going to want to sustain. So, with this in mind I suggest you commit, in the first instance, to giving *The True You Diet* a trial of, say, 30 days. This should be long enough to get real benefit, at which point you can make an informed decision about the longer term.

Assuming that you get beyond this point, it is still important to be aware of some of the major reasons for 'dietary default' – and, more importantly, what can help you counter them.

Why Diets Fail

One obvious reason why individuals end up giving up on a particular diet is that it has failed to have the desired effect. My experience is that what is often going on here is that an individual has embarked on a diet that may have short-term benefits, but is essentially quite the wrong diet for their particular nutritional needs. Now that you are likely to have a better idea of the foods that are right for *you,* you will perhaps be able to see why some of the approaches you have tried in the past have been doomed to fail. Through an identification of your ideal diet, you are now primed to see positive change that is more pervasive and lasting than you may have been accustomed to in the past.

Why Hunger Has No Part to Play in Weight Loss

If one of your primary reasons for buying this book was to lose weight, you may have somewhere tucked away in your subconscious – or possibly even at the forefront of your mind – the notion that success will require you to spend at least some of the day feeling hungry. On some level you may be programmed to believe that in order to shed pounds you simply will not be able to eat food in quantities big enough to fully satisfy your appetite.

While some, including many health professionals, see hunger as a prerequisite to weight loss, I see it as quite the reverse. There is nothing quite like dietary deprivation to sap the resolve. While most of us can put up with this sensation for a few days or even weeks, very, very few will be able to tough it out for any longer. What usually happens is that an individual will end up going back to their original diet, which inevitably brings with it a return of any weight that was lost.

However, in the process of 'going hungry' the body will normally have gone into 'survival mode' and down-tuned its metabolic rate. The metabolic rate may not recover in a timely fashion when fuel intakes increase once more. In one study, the effect of long-term calorie restriction was found to suppress metabolic rate,[1] and this suppression was still found to be significant six months after any dietary restrictions had come to an end. This helps to explain why so many individuals find after a diet that the weight they regain is actually greater than the weight they lost. It is largely because of the unsustainable nature of restrictive regimes and their effect on the metabolism and weight in the long term that you will not find within the pages of this book anything in the way of recommended weights, measures or calorie intakes.

One other reason I have made no limits on intake of permitted foods is that, in my experience, there is usually *no need. The True You Diet* is about fuelling your body with the foods that it 'burns' most efficiently. Give your body the right type of fuel and does it really matter precisely how much of it you give? Going back to the fire analogy we have used earlier in this book, will a bit more wood or coal put on the fire in the evening not have burned by the following morning? Remember, also, we have learned that eating the right foods can actually *stimulate* the metabolism, in a manner similar to the increase in heat and light we get when we fuel a fire appropriately. Get the *type* of fuel right, and *how much* of that fuel we provide for the body is a secondary concern.

Also – and this is very important – my experience is that when individuals eat in accordance with their body's genuine nutritional needs, they almost always eat *less* anyway. One explanation for this is that all three of the core diets in this book will help ensure stability in blood-sugar and insulin levels, which in itself tends to quell an appetite that can run out of control. In addition, the internal processes that regulate how much we eat have some ability to detect when we are giving the body what it really wants and needs. That way, we can keep our internal 'fire' alive with smaller quantities of appropriate fuel, rather than piling in greater quantities of a fuel that stubbornly refuses to really catch alight. The key here is not to concentrate on the quantity of the food you eat, but its *quality*.

There's No Reason to Be Rigid

Quite a lot of people I meet in my personal or professional life have an 'all-or-nothing' mentality when it comes to healthy eating. In other words, either they are sticking assiduously to the letter of the law of some diet, or their diet is all over the place. I wouldn't have written this book if I didn't believe there are some fundamental nutritional rules that need to be borne in mind if we value our health and well-being. However, I don't recommend too strict an approach.

Rather than swinging between dietary extremes, a better long-term approach is to get the bulk of your diet right, and be satisfied with that. This is particularly important when it's difficult to control your diet. For example, if you happened to be staying with friends then it might be considered bad form to dictate what food you are served. You may want to throw the rules out the window when you're on holiday, too. If you're having a business meeting at lunchtime and sandwiches are served, what are you going to do: *starve*?

The important thing here is that you do not let these incidents cloud the bigger picture. Rather than focusing on individual meals, the aim is to keep an overview of the totality of your diet. See whatever you eat in the context of your diet as a whole. It is sometimes worth reminding yourself that it's what you eat *most* of the time, not some of it, that will essentially determine the benefits you get from *The True You Diet* in the long term.

Another thing to keep in mind that might help you take a slightly more relaxed and confident attitude to your eating is that the longer you eat in accordance with your body's needs, the more you can generally 'get away with'. Basically, the more stable your biochemistry is, the more it will take to knock it out of balance. So, to give you an example, after some time of eating in accordance with their needs, 'hunters' often find that the biscuits or chocolate they used to gorge on can now be eaten in moderation without any desire for more. Another example is the 'gatherer' who finds that a weekend 'blow-out' simply does not register on the scales like it may have done in the past.

Changing Times

The ability of the body to adjust and 'right itself' may have other implications, too. For instance, it is possible for individuals to find that their ideal diet can change over time. Because of this possibility, I encourage you to have this at the back of your mind and respond to any signals that your body may be giving you that your dietary needs have changed. One common symptom to look out for here is hunger. Should you find yourself consistently needing more food than is usual for you, then I suggest you tune in to what it is that your body appears to be asking for. 'Hunters', for instance, may feel they need a bit more carbohydrate in the form of some potatoes or brown rice as an accompaniment to a typical meal. For 'gatherers', there may be an increased desire for foods rich in protein and fat, such as meat or eggs.

For some, these shifts can even come and go with the seasons. For example, a 'hunter-gatherer' may find that salads make perfectly satisfying evening meals in the warmer summer months, but that they need more in the way of heartier, heavier food such as stews and casseroles in the winter. There is every possibility that these changing nutritional requirements come, again, from our ancient past when food availability – and therefore suitability – may have changed significantly over the course of the year. This phenomenon is a good argument for eating seasonal produce. This has environmental benefits too, as does eating food sourced as locally as possible.

The Propaganda Problem

Another major reason for 'dietary defaulting' concerns what I regard as nutritional propaganda: dietary advice, information and indoctrination that come from parties more motivated by profit than by your personal health concerns. I mentioned this factor in the Introduction, and in subsequent chapters we have explored a few examples of how it seems we have been fed a lot of rubbish, both literally and metaphorically, in the interests of making money. I have little doubt that soon after putting this book down you will, for instance, read or hear something that alerts you, yet again, to the supposed perils of eating animal fat, while at the same time exalting foods of dubious nutritional value such as wholemeal bread, fat-reduced milk, pre-packaged, processed breakfast cereals with added sugar and salt, margarine and artificial sweeteners.

The reason I want to return to this topic here is that I know from my experience in practice how powerful and pervasive these erroneous messages can be, and how easy it is for some individuals to become insecure about their diet (particularly those eating a fatty 'hunter' diet). That is why I have done my best in this book to set the nutritional record straight through a thorough appraisal of the science. Even armed with this informa-tion it can sometimes take a strong person and quite a degree of conviction to reject, for instance, their doctor's recommendation to eschew red meat and butter because of an 'elevated' cholesterol level. I don't encourage you to reject what health professionals say out of hand. However, I do advise a healthy degree of scepticism.

I am a great believer in individuals being their own advocates. Knowledge is power, as they say, and that is partly why this book takes quite a science-based approach. Reading and inwardly digesting this book will help you discern science fact from science fiction.

And Finally ...

While I believe that research and scientific endeavour can do much to inform us, I know that keeping all this information in our heads and at our fingertips is a challenge in itself. It is my belief, therefore, that for you to have a chance of successfully applying the principles of *The True You Diet* in your life, in the long term it's important for you to have a clear picture in your mind of its basic premise.

And I do mean *picture*. Just conjure up now a picture of our early ances-tors, perhaps sitting around a campfire, feasting on some primal fare. What can you see? Meat? Maybe fish? How about some fruit, vegetable matter and nuts? To most, these images seem utterly plausible. However, you may find it harder to visualize early man and woman tucking into cheese sandwiches, bagels, biscuits, bowls of breakfast cereals and platefuls of pasta, all washed down with an artificially sweetened soft drink. Irrespective of your precise nutritional needs, having this image in your mind will keep you out of a lot of dietary trouble, not just now but for the rest of your life. Whatever new-fangled, highly processed, chemically adulterated, nutritionally bereft foods the food industry dreams up and touts to us, just going back to this ancestral image will help you discern what's healthy from what's not.

As you have made your way through this book, you may have found that the notion of eating in accordance with our ancient diet resonated with an innate wisdom that you feel you've had all along. It's not just *science* that tells us that going back to our nutritional roots is the right path to take, but *common sense*.

Recipes

'Hunter' Recipes

Starters

Chorizo, chestnut, Manchego and coriander salad

Onion soup with beef leftovers and horseradish cream

Smoked duck, rocket, watercress and hazelnut salad

Chicken liver pâté with onion marmalade

Parma ham, rocket and pesto salad

Mains

Beef chilli with avocado salsa

Pork belly with apples, Calvados gravy and curly kale with garlic

Beef with Belgian beer and easy cauliflower goat's cheese

Slow-roast rib of beef with roasted beets

Leg of lamb chermoula with mint, tomato, feta and onion salad

Quick guinea fowl Thai stir-fry with green beans and basil

Caramelized T-bone steaks with haloumi, capers and lime

Starters

Chorizo, Chestnut, Manchego and Coriander Salad

This salad has obvious Spanish influences and is delicious in all seasons. It takes 5 minutes to cook.

Serves 2

8 whole chestnuts (fresh chestnuts in season, but otherwise vacuum-packed chestnuts are fine)

12 thick slices (3mm) chorizo

2 handfuls rocket

I handful coriander leaves

Manchego cheese

olive oil

½ a lemon

Heat a dry pan and add the chestnuts. Cook until golden brown, and then place on a plate. In the same pan and on a medium heat, add the sliced chorizo and cook until golden brown. Build a salad of rocket leaves and sprigs of coriander. Add the chestnuts and the chorizo and place on a serving dish. Top the salad with shavings of Manchego cheese and drizzle with olive oil and lemon juice.

Onion Soup with Beef Leftovers and Horseradish Cream

Serves 4

55g unsalted butter

790g onions, finely sliced

2 cloves garlic, finely chopped

45g plain flour

2 litres beef stock

1 glass (225ml) dry white wine

1 fresh bay leaf

2 sprigs of your favourite fresh herb (rosemary, thyme, marjoram for example)

2 tbs horseradish sauce

110ml double cream

leftover roast beef slices, shredded

Melt the butter in a heavy-based pan and add the onions. Cook over a low heat for 25 minutes or until the onion is golden brown and starting to caramelize. Add the garlic and flour and stir for 2 minutes. Blend in the stock, wine and herbs and simmer for 30 minutes. Remove the herbs and season to taste. Mix the horseradish sauce with the cream and then divide the soup among warmed soup bowls. Top the soup with the shredded roast beef and a teaspoon of the horseradish cream.

Smoked Duck, Rocket, Watercress and Hazelnut Salad

Serves two

2 large handfuls rocket and watercress

2 tbsp hazelnut oil

2 tbsp white wine vinegar

1 tsp Dijon mustard

1 smoked duck breast, cold, cut into 6–8 slices

1 good handful of roasted hazelnuts, roughly chopped

salt and pepper

Place the salad leaves in a bowl and set aside. Heat the hazelnut oil, wine vinegar and mustard in a saucepan for a few minutes until warm. Pour this mixture over the salad leaves, then arrange the duck slices on top. Sprinkle with the roasted hazelnuts and season with salt and pepper.

Chicken Liver Pâté with Onion Marmalade

Serves 6–8

For the pâté

170g unsalted butter, softened

450g trimmed chicken livers (you can soak them in milk for 12 hours before – this helps to mellow any acidity)

1 red onion, finely chopped

2 cloves garlic, finely chopped

1 tbs fresh thyme

1 shot brandy

black pepper

For the marmalade

110g unsalted butter

900g red onions, sliced

2 tbs sugar

salt and pepper

dash red wine vinegar

dash grenadine syrup (optional)

37cl (half-bottle) red wine

To make the pâté, heat a knob of the butter in a frying pan. Add the livers and sauté quickly until golden (3–4 minutes). Place the livers into a food processor. In the same pan add the onion, garlic and thyme until the onion is softened. Add the brandy and black pepper, and deglaze the pan to release the entire pan's flavour. Place in the food processor with the liver and the rest of the butter. Blend to your preferred texture. Cover, cool and refrigerate.

For the marmalade, melt the butter in a saucepan and add the onions. Add the sugar, season well and cover. Simmer for 20 minutes and then add the red wine vinegar, grenadine syrup and red wine. Cook, uncovered, over a low heat for approximately 2 hours until the onions are thick and the juices bubble gently. Cool and refrigerate. The marmalade can be served warm or cold.

Parma Ham, Rocket and Pesto Salad

Serves 2

200g rocket leaves

1 clove garlic

10 tsp extra-virgin olive oil

2 tbs white wine vinegar

110g grated Parmesan

Parma ham

Put the rocket in a food processor with the garlic. Blend until coarse and then add the olive oil, white wine vinegar and Parmesan. Season to taste, then place slices of Parma ham on a platter. Dress the ham with the pesto liberally and then serve.

Mains

Beef Chilli with Avocado Salsa

Serves 6–8

olive oil

2 red onions, chopped

2 cloves garlic, chopped

6 bird's eye chillies, deseeded and chopped

110g portobello mushrooms, chopped

790g best braising steak, thickly sliced

2 tsp ground cumin

2 tsp smoked paprika

1 tsp cayenne pepper

½ cinnamon stick

2 fresh bay leaves

2 tins plum tomatoes

225ml red wine

225ml beef stock

1 tin red kidney beans (drained and rinsed)

30g dark chocolate

salt and pepper

1 ripe avocado

handful fresh coriander

1 lime

crème fraiche

Heat the oil in a heavy-based pan and add three-quarters of the onion until soft. Add the garlic, chillies and mushrooms and cook for 5 minutes. Transfer the mixture to a plate and, in the same pan, brown the meat in batches. Add the onion mixture to the beef, then add the cumin, paprika, cayenne, cinnamon, bay leaves, tomatoes, red wine and beef stock. Bring to the boil and simmer for 1 hour. Add the kidney beans and simmer for a further 30 minutes. Stir in the chocolate. Season and add more fresh chilli if required.

Chop the avocado and mix with coriander leaves, lime juice and the remaining red onion. Serve the chilli in bowls topped with the salsa and a tablespoon of crème fraiche.

Pork Belly with Apples, Calvados Gravy and Curly Kale with Garlic

Serves 4

1 whole pork belly, boned, scored and well seasoned with salt and pepper

pork belly bones

2 onions, sliced

2 sprigs rosemary

2 sprigs thyme

2 fresh bay leaves

1 tbs peppercorns

450ml water

4 Granny Smith apples, peeled and quartered

30g butter

2 tsp brown sugar

1 tbs Calvados

2 tbs crème fraiche

1 clove garlic, crushed

curly kale, washed and sliced

2 tbs water

In a deep roasting dish, place the well-seasoned pork belly on top of the bones, onions, rosemary, thyme, bay leaves and peppercorns. Add water to the roasting dish and cover with a tent of foil (make sure that the foil is not touching the meat). Place in a pre-heated oven at 300°F/150°C/Gas Mark 2 for 6 hours.

After 6 hours, remove the pork belly from the roasting dish and place on a separate oven tray. Turn up the oven to 425°F/220°C/Gas Mark 7. Strain the juices from the meat into a jug and skim the fat from the top of the liquid once it has settled. Return the pork to the oven for 25 minutes. Remove the pork from the oven and rest for 15 minutes.

While resting the pork, sauté the apples in butter in a frying pan for a minute, add the sugar and cook until the apples are caramelized. Remove and keep warm. Add the Calvados to the pan and then the strained and skimmed juices from the meat. Add the crème fraiche and stir to make the gravy. Reduce the gravy on a medium heat for 10 minutes to a rich consistency. In a large saucepan, sauté the garlic until softened and add the seasoned curly kale and 2 tablespoons of water. Heat for 2 minutes until the kale is soft and tender. Chop the pork into large pieces and serve with the curly kale and the apples. Pass the gravy round.

Beef with Belgian Beer and Easy Cauliflower Goat's Cheese

For this dish a strong beer like a Leffe Dark is recommended.

Serves 6–8

For the beef

unsalted butter

170g bacon lardons

900g red onions, thinly sliced

1 tbs brown sugar

75g plain flour

salt and pepper

2kg best braising steak, cut into generous chunks

110ml red wine

560ml Leffe Dark Beer

1 bouquet garni

For the cauliflower cheese

1 head cauliflower, trimmed and cut into small florets

280g cream cheese

1 tsp French mustard

110g strong goat's cheese, cut into small pieces, without rind

salt and pepper

55g goat's cheddar cheese

3 tbs French mustard

handful flat-leaf parsley, chopped

watercress

Melt a knob of soft, unsalted butter in a large oven-proof casserole pot and fry the lardons until brown. Remove the lardons, add the onions to the pot and cook slowly for 25 minutes until golden brown. Increase the heat, add the sugar and cook until caramelized. Remove the onions and set aside.

Season the flour with salt and pepper and coat the steak in the flour. Brown the beef in batches and, once finished, deglaze the dish with the red wine, and then add half the beer. Bring to the boil and add the bouquet garni. Add the remaining beer, the beef, the onions and the lardons. Cover the dish with foil, sealing the edges, and put the lid on the casserole dish. Bake at 325°F/160°C/Gas Mark 3 for 2½ hours.

After 2 hours you are ready to make the cauliflower goat's cheese.

Bring 5cm-depth of water to the boil in a saucepan, add the cauliflower and cook for about 8 minutes, or until tender. Drain and return the cauliflower to the pan. Mix the cream cheese and mustard with the cauliflower, then stir in the goat's cheese. Season with a little salt if necessary and plenty of pepper. Pour the mixture into a shallow gratin dish, then cover with the goat's cheddar. Place under a preheated hot grill for 10–15 minutes, or until the top is golden brown and the inside hot and bubbling.

Bring out the beef and sprinkle with the parsley. Serve with the cauliflower cheese and a watercress salad.

Slow-roast Rib of Beef with Roasted Beets

Serves 6–8

2 large onions, thickly sliced

5 sprigs thyme

5 sprigs rosemary

3kg piece of well-hung forerib of beef (from a butcher) on the bone

85g unsalted butter, softened

3 tbs French mustard

salt and pepper

8 medium-sized raw beetroots

Pre-heat the oven to 450°F/230°C/Gas Mark 8. Put the onion slices in the middle of a roasting dish, to act like a natural trivet. Place the herb sprigs across the onion and place the beef on top. Mix the butter and mustard and spread half the mix all over the beef. Season the beef well with salt and pepper.

Wash the beetroot and position around the beef. Transfer the dish to the oven and roast, uncovered, for 25 minutes. Reduce the heat to 325°F/160°C/Gas Mark 3 and roast for 35 minutes per kilogram. Turn the oven off and put the other half of the mustard butter on the beef. Leave the oven door open and leave the beef to rest for 15 minutes.

Remove the beef, onion and herbs from the dish and heat the juices on the stove top, seasoning to taste. Carve the beef and put slices on a warm platter with the beets. Pour the gravy over the beef and beets and serve with hot horseradish sauce.

Leg of Lamb Chermoula with Mint, Tomato, Feta and Onion Salad

Chermoula is a blend of spices and tastes that derive from Mediterranean Africa. Working with lamb, these tastes are a wonderful combination and are offset by the sharpness of a feta salad.

Serves 6–8

1 tbs cumin seeds

1 tbs black peppercorns

1 tsp chilli powder

1 tbs smoked paprika

1 tbs coriander seeds

juice of 2 lemons

3 cloves garlic, crushed

5 tbs extra-virgin olive oil

1 bunch coriander

2kg leg of lamb

6 plum tomatoes

1 slab feta cheese

2 red onions, finely sliced

1 handful fresh mint, finely chopped

Take the cumin seeds, black peppercorns, chilli powder, smoked paprika and coriander seeds and toast in a dry pan until the spices are smoking lightly. Grind the spice mixture in a pestle and mortar and put in a food processor. Add the lemon juice, garlic, olive oil and coriander to the food processor and blend until it becomes a coarse paste.

Preheat the oven to 425°F/220°C/Gas Mark 7. With a sharp knife, cut small deep slits in the top and sides of the lamb. With the back of a spoon rub the paste all over the lamb and then use your hands to spread the paste and make sure all the lamb is covered.

Put the lamb bone-side down in a deep roasting dish and put on the top shelf of the oven. Bake for 10 minutes, then baste and return to the oven. Reduce the temperature to 300°F/150°C/Gas Mark 2. Bake the lamb for 3 hours 30 minutes, basting every 15–20 minutes. Remove the lamb from the oven and rest for 15 minutes.

While the lamb is resting, slice the tomatoes and add to the crumbled feta and sliced onions. Sprinkle the salad with fresh mint leaves and drizzle with olive oil and lemon juice. Carve the meat and serve with the salad.

Quick Guinea Fowl Thai Stir-fry with Green Beans and Basil

This dish also works well with chicken, pork or beef.

Serves 4

1 tbs vegetable oil

2 tbs red curry paste

2 guinea fowl fillets, thinly sliced

110g fine green beans

110ml coconut milk

55g chopped spring onions

1 tbs lime juice

1 tbs fish sauce

1 tsp palm sugar

30g basil leaves

1 red chilli, thinly sliced

Heat a wok over a high heat, adding the oil and curry paste. Cook for 1 minute. Add the guinea fowl and cook for 2–3 minutes. Add the fine green beans and coconut milk and cook for 1–2 minutes. Stir in the spring onions. Finally add the lime juice, fish sauce and sugar and stir in. Serve in warm bowls and garnish with basil leaves and chilli.

Caramelized T-bone Steaks with Haloumi, Capers and Lime

Other good cuts for this dish include sirloin, fillet or rib-eye.

Serves 2

2 cloves garlic, chopped

2 tbs extra-virgin olive oil

1 tbs fresh basil, chopped

1 tbs brown sugar

1 tsp French mustard

2 tbs balsamic vinegar

2 400g well-seasoned T-bone steaks

4 slices Haloumi cheese

2 tbs capers, crushed

juice of ½ a lime

pepper

Preheat a barbecue or griddle pan to medium-high heat. Combine the garlic, oil, basil, sugar, mustard and vinegar in a bowl. Add the steaks and marinade for 5 minutes. Cook the steaks to your liking. Rest the steaks for 2 minutes.

While the meat is resting, heat a non-stick frying pan over a medium heat. Add the haloumi and cook for 1 minute on each side. Serve the haloumi on a plate with the crushed capers, lime juice and a drizzle of olive oil. Place the steaks on top of the haloumi and season with pepper.

'Hunter-Gatherer' Recipes

Starters

Thai chicken soup

Pea and ham soup

Chicken soup

Smoked haddock and coconut soup

Grilled sardines with tomato and preserved lemon salad

Mains

Rabbit with prunes

Salmon Niçoise

Venison casserole

Roast chicken

Shepherd's pie with minted mushy peas

Rabbit stew

Frittata

Starters

Thai Chicken Soup

Serves 2

560ml chicken stock

335ml coconut milk

2 stalks lemongrass, halved and bruised in a pestle and mortar

2 green chillies, sliced

2 chicken breasts, very thinly sliced

juice of ½ a lime

2 tsp Thai fish sauce

1 tsp palm sugar

coriander leaves

basil leaves

1 red chilli, deseeded and sliced

Place the stock, coconut milk, lemongrass and chillies in a pan and bring to the boil. Simmer for 3 minutes, add the chicken and cook for 3 minutes. Add the lime juice, the fish sauce and the palm sugar. Serve the soup in bowls with fresh coriander, basil leaves and red chilli.

Pea and Ham Soup

Serves 2

200g good-quality bacon or ham, preferably in one piece

2 tbs olive oil

30g butter

2 onions, finely chopped

1 large potato, chopped into 2cm chunks

3 cloves garlic, finely chopped

800g frozen peas

stock or water

salt and pepper

Remove the hard, outer part of the bacon rind and cut the bacon up into small pieces. Gently fry in the olive oil until cooked but not too crispy. Remove from the pan and set aside. Put the butter in the pan, add the onions and sauté over a gentle heat for 5 minutes, stirring from time to time. Add the potato chunks and continue to cook and stir for a further 5 minutes or until the onions are translucent. Add the garlic and cook gently for a minute. Add the peas and mix well. Cook for a couple of minutes.

Cover with stock/water and bring to the boil, then lower the temperature and allow to simmer gently for 30 minutes. Blend until smooth, adding more water if necessary. Add the bacon/ham and stir. Add salt and pepper to taste.

Variation

Try making this with dried split green peas (which have been soaked and cooked) instead of the peas for a more substantial soup.

Chicken Soup

Serves 2–4

For the stock

1 onion

1 carrot

2 sticks celery

parsley and thyme

bay leaf

1 chicken (preferably organic or at least free range)

For the soup

olive oil and/or dripping

2 onions, finely chopped

2 sticks celery, thinly sliced

3 carrots, cut into ½cm slices cut on a slant

4 small potatoes, thickly sliced (optional)

100g green lentils

stock or water

salt and pepper

pieces of chicken left over from a roast bird (see below)

sprig of fresh thyme or a pinch of dried thyme

large handful finely chopped parsley

Remove all the useable meat from the chicken and set aside. Then use the carcass to make a stock.

If you have the giblets from the bird, use these too.

Place all the ingredients (except the chicken meat) in a pan, cover with water and bring to the boil. Reduce the heat and simmer gently for 1 hour. Strain into a bowl and allow to cool.

Remove all the fat from the surface of the stock and discard. If you don't want to use the stock immediately you can cool it and then freeze it.

Pour the olive oil into a large, heavy-bottomed pan, add the onions and cook over a medium heat, stirring occasionally. Add the celery, the carrots and finally the potatoes. Cook, stirring occasionally for 10 minutes until the vegetables are beginning to soften. Add the lentils and stir well. At this point add the stock if you are using it, otherwise almost cover the vegetables with boiling water and season. Cover and simmer gently for about 30 minutes or until the vegetables are tender, stirring occasionally. Add the pieces of chicken and heat through for another 15 minutes. Check the seasoning and add the thyme and parsley just before you serve the soup.

Variations

Other meats can be used in this soup, such as pheasant or turkey. Try other vegetables in the soup: finely shredded spring greens, leeks, broccoli or green beans or finely diced swede. You can also vary the pulses: try haricot beans, red lentils or Puy lentils for example, or omit them altogether.

Smoked Haddock and Coconut Soup

Serves 4

280g naturally smoked haddock (not the bright yellow kind!)

water

dash of olive oil

170g onions, finely chopped

450g carrots, finely diced

110g celery, finely chopped

white part of 1 small leek, well washed and finely chopped

½ tin coconut milk

salt and pepper

handful coriander

Place the haddock in a wide-bottomed pan and scantily cover with water. Simmer until the fish is cooked and flaky, but do not overcook. This should take 5–10 minutes. Leave to cool then remove the fish carefully from the cooking liquid and keep the liquid. Put the oil in a large pan, add the onions and let them sweat over a medium heat, stirring to prevent them catching on the bottom of the pan. After about 5 minutes, add the rest of the vegetables and stir until they start to become tender.

Add the cooking liquid from the fish and enough water to nearly cover the vegetables. Bring to the boil, then lower the heat and simmer gently for 20 minutes. Remove the skin from the fish and flake the fish into small bite-sized pieces, removing any bones as you find them. Add the fish and the coconut milk to the soup and heat through gently. Season to taste. Add a good handful of finely chopped coriander to the soup and serve.

Grilled Sardines with Tomato and Preserved Lemon Salad

Serves 1

2 fresh sardines

salt and black pepper

2 ripe plum tomatoes or 1 beef tomato, sliced

1 preserved lemon, sliced

1 tbs fresh coriander

olive oil

lemon juice

Preheat a grill to high (you can use a barbecue if preferred). Season with salt and black pepper and place under the grill for 3–4 minutes each side, until cooked. As the sardines are cooking, make the salad. Arrange on a plate the sliced tomatoes and preserved lemon, sprinkle with chopped coriander and drizzle with olive oil and lemon juice. Arrange the cooked sardines on top and serve.

Mains

Rabbit with Prunes

Serves 2–4

5 tbs olive oil

3 small onions, halved and thinly sliced

2 sticks celery, finely diced

675g carrots, cut lengthways and then on a slant into ½cm slices

1 whole head of garlic, peeled and thinly sliced

1.1kg rabbit or hare, jointed. You can ask the butcher to do this.

170g stoned prunes

500ml decent red wine

1 tin plum tomatoes, peeled and chopped

2 bay leaves

½ dozen sprigs fresh thyme or a couple of pinches of dried thyme

salt and pepper

Pour the olive oil into a large pan. A cast-iron pan that will go into the oven is ideal, otherwise one that will comfortably hold all the ingredients. Place on a medium heat on the stovetop. Add the onions and stir occasionally to prevent them from sticking. Add the celery, then the carrots and garlic. Keep cooking and stirring the vegetables. Heat a little oil in another (heavy-bottomed) frying pan to medium-high and brown the rabbit pieces well, in batches, transferring to the vegetables as you go along.

When you have finished browning the meat, set the frying pan aside. You will need all the meaty residue it contains in a minute. Add the prunes. Stir and cook on a gentle heat for 10 minutes. Return the second frying pan to the heat and, when warm, carefully pour in the red wine and scrape all the little bits of meat and juice off the pan and mix with the wine.

Pour the wine over the meat and vegetables. Then add the tomatoes, the bay leaves and the thyme and season. Bring to the boil and simmer gently for 3 hours or until the meat is meltingly tender, checking from time to time. If the pan that you are using will go into the oven, then cook in the oven at about 300°F/150°C/Gas Mark 2 – but check to see that it is just simmering, no more. Check the seasoning before serving.

This dish goes very well with Puy lentils, but can also be served with some plain boiled or mashed potatoes and plenty of steamed green vegetables.

Salmon Niçoise

Serves 4

For the dressing

1 large clove garlic, finely chopped

1 heaped tsp wholegrain mustard

juice of 2 limes

8 tbs olive oil

salt and pepper

2 tbs finely chopped parsley

For the salad

8 small new potatoes or waxy salad potatoes

water

a little butter

salt and pepper

2 tbs finely chopped parsley

450g French green beans (haricots verts), topped and tailed

olive oil

4 eggs

4 salmon fillets – preferably wild or organic

rocket or other salad greens – enough to cover the plate you're using

⅓ of a jar of caper berries

Mix all the dressing ingredients together in a clean jam jar. Put the lid on and shake well. Wash the potatoes and place in a pan. Cover with water and bring to the boil. Lower the heat and simmer until tender. Drain. Toss in a little butter, salt and pepper and finely chopped parsley. If you have a steamer that fits onto your pan, steam the green beans above the potatoes. Otherwise, place the beans in a pan with a little cold water, bring to the boil, lower the heat, cover and simmer until just tender. Drain. Toss in olive oil, salt and pepper.

Place the eggs in a pan, cover with water, bring to the boil and simmer for 5 minutes. Take off the heat but leave in the water for a further 10 minutes. Pour out the hot water and run cold water into the pan until cool. Leave the eggs in the cold water for 5 minutes, then peel and quarter. Preheat your grill. Place the salmon fillets onto a lightly oiled, shallow baking tray and cook the salmon for about 5 minutes – a little longer if necessary but do not overcook. When you insert a sharp knife into the fish it should look flaky all the way through.

To assemble the salad use a large platter or plate and cover with the rocket or salad leaves of your choice. Grind some pepper and drizzle a little olive oil over the leaves. Put the potatoes onto the leaves, then add the green beans, making sure they are evenly distributed over the plate. Nestle the eggs in amongst the beans and potatoes. Carefully remove the skin from the salmon, break into large chunks and arrange on the salad – or leave whole if you prefer. Shake the dressing and pour all over the salad, then add the caper berries.

Serve immediately.

Variations

You may, of course, add any other salad vegetable that you like: cherry tomatoes, strips of red pepper, slithers of fennel, for example. Also consider the addition of olives. Try coriander instead of parsley in the dressing, and scatter a handful of chopped coriander over the whole dish before serving.

Venison Casserole

This is even better the next day, so you might want to make double quantities!

Serves 4

olive oil

2 large onions, coarsely chopped

2 sticks celery, finely chopped

4 carrots, cut into ½cm discs on a slant

4 cloves garlic, finely chopped

1kg venison stewing steak cut into 2½cm chunks and dried on kitchen roll if necessary. It is essential for the meat to be dry in order to brown well. You can use any good cut of venison here. The better the cut, the more tender the meat.

⅔ bottle decent red wine

1 can chopped peeled plum tomatoes

2 bay leaves

4 juniper berries, crushed open

a couple of sprigs of fresh thyme or a pinch or two of dried thyme

salt and pepper

Pour a generous amount of olive oil into a large pan. A cast-iron pan that will go into the oven is ideal; otherwise one that will comfortably hold all the ingredients. Place on a medium heat. Add the onions and stir occasionally to prevent them from sticking. Add the finely chopped celery, then add the carrots and garlic.

Keep cooking and stirring the vegetables while you place a little olive oil into a different, heavy-bottomed frying pan. Heat to medium-high and brown the venison steak chunks well in batches, transferring to the vegetables as you go along.

When you have finished browning the meat set the frying pan aside. You will need all the meaty residue therein in a minute. Stir the meat and vegetables and cook on a gentle heat for 10 minutes. Return the second frying pan to the heat and, when warm, carefully pour in the red wine and scrape all the little bits of meat and juice off the pan and mix with the wine. Pour the wine over the vegetables and the meat. Then add the tomatoes, the bay leaves, the juniper berries and the thyme and season.

Bring to the boil and simmer gently for 3 hours or until the meat is meltingly tender, checking from time to time. If the pan that you are using will go into the oven then cook in the oven at about 300°F/150°C/Gas Mark 2, but check to see that it is just simmering. Check the seasoning before serving.

Serve on its own or with Puy lentils, potatoes, mashed potatoes and celeriac, steamed broccoli, braised cabbage, steamed green beans, etc.

Roast Chicken

Serves 4–6

1 lemon

1 whole large chicken

I bunch tarragon

salt and pepper

Halve the lemon and push it inside the chicken with the tarragon.

Roast the whole chicken in a preheated oven at about 400°F/200°C/Gas Mark 6. Allow about 20 minutes for 500g of bird, plus another 20 minutes.

Serve with green vegetables and some roast parsnips and/or potatoes.

Shepherd's Pie with Minted Mushy Peas

Serves 4–6

olive oil

1 large onion, finely chopped

450g minced lamb – from a roasted shoulder or roasted leg

1 tsp plain flour

2 fresh bay leaves

2 sprigs rosemary

280ml lamb stock

225ml red wine

2 tbs Worcestershire sauce

salt and black pepper

675g potatoes (Desiree or King Edward)

85g butter

1 egg yolk

1 tin mushy peas

1 tbs chopped mint leaves

1 tsp white wine vinegar

You have two ways of sourcing the lamb mince for this dish. If you're in a hurry you can buy fresh lamb mince from the butcher. On the other hand, you can roast a shoulder of lamb at your convenience and then both mince the meat and reserve the juices as stock.

In a large non-stick casserole dish, heat 1 tbs of olive oil. Add the onion and cook for 5 minutes. Meanwhile, in a separate large frying pan heat a little olive oil and fry the mince up evenly until browned. While the meat is frying, break up any lumps with the back of the spoon. Stir the onions in the casserole dish, add the flour and stir. Mix well and add the bay leaves and rosemary; stir. To the onion mix add the meat, stock, half the wine and the Worcestershire sauce. Deglaze the frying pan with the other half of the wine and add to the casserole dish. Bring the casserole dish to the boil, adding a pinch of salt and pepper, and let simmer for about 1 hour.

Boil the potatoes, sieve and put into a bowl. Add the butter and egg yolk, and mash together. Season with salt and black pepper. Spread the mash over the meat mixture, smooth over and mark with a spatula. Put the dish into the oven at 375°F/190°C/Gas Mark 5 until it is bubbling and golden – usually 45 minutes.

Warm the mushy peas with chopped mint leaves and vinegar, and serve the dish.

Rabbit Stew

This is a traditional Maltese recipe.

Serves 4–6

1 rabbit (cut into 6 pieces)

1 tbs olive oil

2 onions, chopped

6 garlic cloves

3 large tomatoes, peeled and chopped

3 potatoes, peeled and quartered

225ml red wine

2 tsp tomato paste

225g peas

2 bay leaves

mixed herbs

salt and pepper

Fry the rabbit in olive oil until slightly brown in a casserole dish or large saucepan. Add the onions, garlic, tomatoes and potatoes. Pour some of the wine over. Add the tomato paste, peas and bay leaves. If you have the kidney and liver from the rabbit, add these too (if desired!). Bring to a boil and simmer for about 1½ hours on a low-medium heat. Season to taste. Add more wine if the sauce begins to dry up.

When ready, serve with some green vegetables such as steamed cabbage.

Frittata

A frittata is basically a thick omelette with a filling cooked in a non-stick frying pan.

Serves 2–3

1 large onion, finely chopped

olive oil

4–6 rashers of good-quality bacon, with hard edge of rinds removed, cut into 1cm strips

225g broccoli, cut into small florets

6 medium eggs

salt and pepper

Sauté the onion in the oil with the bacon over a medium heat in a non-stick frying pan, stirring from time to time to prevent them browning. Steam the broccoli for 5 minutes until almost tender, but not soft. Add the broccoli to the bacon and stir for a couple of minutes, then tip into a bowl. Wipe the frying pan.

Crack the eggs into a bowl with generous grindings of pepper and a little salt, and beat with a fork until well blended. Place the non-stick frying pan on a medium heat and pour in 2 tbs of olive oil. Tip the broccoli mixture into the eggs and combine.

Pour this into the warm frying pan and leave for a few seconds; as the eggs start to cook, carefully, using a heat-resistant spatula, lift the egg mixture so that uncooked mixture can slide underneath. Do this all the way around the pan and in the middle too. Don't worry if you seem to be stirring or nudging the eggs gently. The aim is to let the frittata cook enough, without burning on the bottom, so that you can tip it over.

Do this for a minute or so until you feel that the eggs are starting to solidify, then stop – you don't want to end up with scrambled eggs! Every now and then give the pan a little shake to keep the eggs free of the bottom. If necessary change the position of the pan on the ring if you think that the eggs are cooking unevenly.

After a few minutes, when the frittata looks solid enough, take the pan off the heat, give it a shake to make sure that the eggs aren't sticking, and place a plate over it. Wearing oven gloves, clamp the plate firmly over the pan and, very carefully but quite swiftly, invert the pan and the plate so that the frittata ends up on the plate. Take great care, as the top of the frittata will still be a little bit runny. Put another tablespoon of oil into the pan and slide the frittata back in.

Gently shake the pan back and forth a few times to ensure the eggs cook evenly and don't stick to the pan.

Cook for another 5 minutes or so until cooked through. (If you don't fancy this method, instead of turning the frittata over, you could pop it under a pre-heated grill to finish off the cooking.)

Delicious hot or at room temperature.

Variations

You can use all sorts of things for the filling: wilted spinach and potato (preboiled and diced); roast tomatoes and basil; peas, ham and potatoes; onions, sliced sausage and potatoes; sautéed courgettes, sundried tomatoes and basil; smoked haddock and so on. It is a notable vehicle for using up decanted leftovers in the fridge. Also an excellent addition to a packed lunch box or picnic.

Serve with salads of all kinds including bean salads. Try to use a salad that complements the frittata. For example, if you are using tomatoes in the frittata, then you might want to choose a green salad.

'Gatherer' Recipes

Starters

Dahl and coconut soup

Hummus with a twist

Aubergine, tomato, onion and goat's cheese towers

Black-eyed beans and cumin pâté with cucumber raitha

Green split pea and mint soup

Mains

Mexican pie

Indonesian-style vegetables

Bean nut roast with pease pudding

Winter crumble

Spinach paneer with basmati rice and cashew nuts

Monk fish with ginger and lime

Starters

Dahl and Coconut Soup

Serves 4

225g red lentils

675ml water

salt and pepper

1 tsp black mustard seed

splash of oil

1 onion, sliced

2 cloves garlic, crushed

1 green chilli, crushed

30g root ginger, finely chopped

1 tsp ground cumin

½ tsp turmeric

¼ tsp chilli powder

1 tsp garam masala

1 tsp tomato paste

300ml coconut milk

1 tbs chopped coriander

Place the lentils and water in a saucepan. Bring to the boil; reduce heat to a very slow simmer. Cook for about 20 minutes, stirring occasionally and adding more water if necessary to give a soft but not too thick sauce. Season with salt and pepper and put aside.

While the lentils are cooking, in a saucepan add the mustard seed to a splash of hot oil, cook for 1 minute and then add the onion, garlic, chilli, ginger and spices. Cook on a low heat until the mixture is soft.

Stir in the tomato paste and coconut milk and cook gently for 10 minutes. Using an electric hand blender, puree the soup, keeping the texture fairly coarse. Season with fresh coriander.

Serve hot.

Hummus with a Twist

Serves 6–8

450g dried chickpeas soaked overnight

85g green olives, pips removed

85g sundried tomatoes

3 cloves garlic, crushed

1 small fresh green chilli, finely chopped

juice of 1 large lemon

5 tbs tahini

4 tbs olive oil or oil from sundried tomatoes

¼ tsp fresh chilli powder

560ml water from soaked chickpeas

1 tsp ground cumin

salt and ground black pepper

Drain and wash the chickpeas, place in a pan of water, bring to a boil and simmer for 1 hour until soft. Drain and save the liquid.

While the chickpeas are boiling, place the olives, sundried tomatoes, garlic and chilli in a food processor and blend, gradually adding in the saved chickpea liquid and lemon juice until smooth.

Add the tahini and oil and blend, adding more liquid if needed. Add the ground cumin and season.

Serve with vegetable crudités.

Aubergine, Tomato, Onion and Goat's Cheese Towers

Serves 4

1 aubergine, sliced into rounds

salt

2 red onions, cut into rings

2 tomatoes, skinned and sliced

olive oil for brushing

5 tbs olive oil

1 clove garlic, chopped

4 leaves basil, chopped

salt and pepper

2 shallots, thinly sliced

1 tsp tomato paste

1 x 400g tinned chopped tomatoes

200g goat's cheese, sliced

Slice the aubergine, sprinkle with salt and leave for half an hour to allow the bitter juices to drain. Wash and pat dry.

Place aubergine, onions and tomatoes on a baking tray, lightly brush with oil.

Prepare marinade of oil, garlic, basil and salt and pepper.

Marinade aubergine, onions and tomatoes.

To prepare the sauce, sauté the shallots in a splash of oil until soft, stir in tomato paste and tinned tomatoes.

Using a hand blender, process the sauce to a smooth consistency, adding a little water if necessary. Season.

On a baking tray, create four towers by layering the aubergine, tomatoes, onions and goat's cheese, then repeat once more, finishing with goat's cheese.

Place the tray in a preheated oven at 180°C/350°F/Gas Mark 4 for 10 to 15 minutes.

To serve, place towers on a pool of sauce on a plate.

Black-eyed Beans and Cumin Pâté with Cucumber Raitha

Serves 4

For the pâté

splash of oil

½ tsp whole cumin seeds

1 onion, chopped

2 cloves garlic, crushed

1 tsp garam masala

1 tsp ground cumin

60ml vegetable stock

170g dried black-eyed beans soaked overnight, drained, brought to a boil and simmered for 20–30 minutes until soft

2 tbs chopped coriander

salt and ground black pepper

For the raitha

110ml goat's yoghurt

¼ cucumber, peeled and grated

½ tsp chopped fresh mint

salt and ground black pepper

Heat the oil in a saucepan and fry the cumin seeds for a minute, stirring; add onions and garlic and sauté for 2–3 minutes until soft. Add the garam masala and ground cumin and cook for a further minute.

Stir in the stock and cooked beans, bring to the boil and simmer for 10 minutes, then allow to cool slightly.

Put the mixture in a food processor and blend. Add the fresh coriander and seasonings and blend for 30 seconds until smooth.

Grease and line the base of a loaf tin and fill with the mixture, pressing down firmly and levelling the surface with the back of a spoon.

Cook in a preheated oven at 200°C/400°F/Gas Mark 6 for 30 minutes or until firm to the touch.

Allow the pâté to cool, then refrigerate.

For the cucumber raitha, mix all the ingredients together.

Serve the pâté sliced with raitha and salad leaves.

Green Split Pea and Mint Soup

Serves 4

55g butter

1 onion, finely chopped

1 clove garlic, crushed

1 small leek, finely sliced

2 sticks celery, sliced

3–4 stalks thyme picked off the stalks and chopped

450g green split peas, soaked for 1 hour, washed and drained

1 litre vegetable stock

6–8 stalks fresh mint picked off the stalks

salt and pepper

In a pan, melt the butter and fry the onion, garlic, leek, celery and thyme until soft.

Add the split peas, stock and mint, bring to the boil and simmer for 20–30 minutes until soft. Take off the stove.

Using an electric hand blender, process until smooth and season.

Mains

Mexican Pie

Serves 4

olive oil

½ tsp chilli powder

2 tsp ground coriander

1 onion, finely chopped

2 cloves garlic, finely chopped

1 red chilli, finely chopped

2 sticks celery, finely chopped

1 tbs tomato puree

1 x 400g tin chopped tomatoes

1 x 400g tin red kidney beans

salt and pepper

450g broccoli cut into florets

1 red pepper, diced

1 green pepper, diced

450g sweet potatoes cut into bite-sized pieces

225g fresh spinach, stalks removed

450ml vegetable stock

110g polenta

55g butter

2 eggs, beaten

Add the oil and spices to a frying pan, warm, then fry the onion, garlic, chilli and celery until soft.

Add the tomato puree, tomatoes and beans. Season.

Bring to the boil, add the broccoli, peppers, sweet potatoes and spinach, and simmer on a low heat.

Meanwhile, bring the stock to a boil in a saucepan. Very gradually add in the polenta, stirring until thickened.

Mix in half the butter, remove from the heat and leave to cool slightly.

Fold in the eggs and season.

Transfer the vegetables into a suitable ovenproof pie dish. Spoon in the polenta.

Bake in a pre-heated oven at 180°C/350°F/Gas Mark 4 for 30–40 minutes until firm and golden. Dot with the remaining butter.

Serve hot.

Indonesian Style Vegetables

Serves 4

2 tbs peanut oil

1 onion, finely chopped

1 green chilli, finely chopped

2 cloves garlic, crushed

½ tsp root ginger, finely chopped

1 tbs tomato puree

1 x 280g jar peanut butter

560ml vegetable stock

salt and ground black pepper

2 carrots, sliced into thin batons

1 small cauliflower, cut into florets

1 small aubergine, diced

8 baby sweet corn, sliced in half lengthways

2 courgettes, sliced diagonally

110g sugar snap peas

2 tbs olive or toasted sesame oil

2 tbs sesame seeds

juice of 1 lemon

2 tbs chopped coriander

rice noodles

In the peanut oil, fry the onion, chilli, garlic and ginger until soft. Add the tomato puree, peanut butter and stock, stirring until the peanut butter has melted. Season and allow to simmer. Using a wok, stir-fry the carrots, cauliflower, aubergine, sweet corn, courgettes and sugar snap peas in hot olive or sesame oil, keeping them firm. Season.

Add the vegetables to the sauce, simmer and finish by adding sesame seeds, lemon juice and coriander.

Serve on a bed of rice noodles cooked according to the packet instructions.

Bean Nut Roast with Pease Pudding

Serves 4–6

170g aduki beans, soaked overnight

140g green lentils soaked for 1 hour

2 onions, finely chopped

140g chopped mixed nuts

110g haloumi cheese, grated

1 tbs chopped parsley

3 eggs

salt and ground black pepper

30g butter

200g yellow split peas soaked for 1 hour, drained and brought to boil in fresh water then simmered for 20–30 minutes until tender; drained again

Drain aduki beans and bring to a boil in fresh water for 10 minutes, then simmer for 20–30 minutes; drain.

Wash and drain the lentils and bring to a boil in fresh water. Simmer for 20 minutes until tender and drain.

Mash the beans and lentils together and mix in one of the chopped onions.

Add the nuts, cheese and parsley. Beat two of the eggs and add in. Season.

Grease and line the base of a loaf tin and fill with the mixture. Press down firmly and put aside.

Fry the other onion in butter until soft, add the peas and third beaten egg and season.

Transfer to a buttered ovenproof dish

Bake the nut roast and pease pudding in a pre-heated oven at 190°C/375°F/Gas Mark 5 for 30 minutes or until set.

Serve nut roast and pease pudding with vegetables of your choice and onion gravy.

Winter Crumble

Serves 4–6

225g butter beans, soaked overnight

water

170g butter

1 onion, finely chopped

1 stick celery, sliced

2 carrots, grated

2 tomatoes, diced

1 tsp fresh thyme, chopped

560ml vegetable stock

1 tbs tomato puree

1 tsp mustard powder

225g leeks, sliced

225g parsnips, cut into chunks

225g turnips, peeled and diced

110g swede, peeled and diced

225g small Brussels sprouts with outer leaves removed

110g oatmeal

85g ground almonds

85g chopped walnuts

85g chopped hazelnuts

salt and pepper

1 tbs caraway seeds

Drain the butter beans and bring to a boil in fresh water for 10 minutes. Simmer for 30 minutes until soft. Drain and put aside.

Melt 55g of the butter in a pan, add the onion, celery, one of the carrots, the tomatoes and the thyme; cook until soft.

Turn down the heat and add the stock, puree and mustard powder and simmer.

In another 55g of the butter stir-fry the leeks, parsnips, turnips, swede and the other carrot.

Blanch the sprouts in boiling water. Cook so the vegetables still have some bite to them.

Combine the vegetables and butter beans with the sauce. Season and simmer. Turn into a suitable ovenproof dish.

For the crumble, mix together the oatmeal, ground almonds and nuts. Season. Mix in the last third of the butter (55g) until the mixture resembles coarse breadcrumbs.

Sprinkle the crumble over the vegetables and finish with caraway seeds.

Bake in a preheated oven at 190°C/375°F/Gas Mark 5 for about 20–25 minutes until crisp.

Serve hot with steamed cabbage.

Spinach Paneer with Basmati Rice and Cashew Nuts

Serves 4

4 tbs olive oil

¾ tsp chilli powder

1½ tsp ground cumin

1½ tsp ground coriander

1½ tsp garam masala

¾ tsp turmeric

salt and pepper

1 packet of paneer (Indian cheese), cubed

55g butter

1 onion, finely sliced

110g raw cashew nuts

170g brown basmati rice

675ml boiling water

¼ tsp fenugreek seeds

1 clove garlic, chopped

1 small green chilli, finely chopped

½ tsp root ginger, chopped

400g leaf spinach

2 tbs chopped coriander

1 shallot, sliced

For the marinade, mix the olive oil, and half a teaspoon each of the chilli powder, ground cumin, ground coriander and garam masala, a quarter teaspoon of the turmeric and salt and pepper together. Add the cubed paneer and put aside.

For the rice, heat the butter in a pan, add half the onion and cook until soft. Add the cashew nuts and drained basmati rice. Cook for a further 5 minutes, stirring. Season.

Add boiling water and simmer gently for 20–30 minutes until all the water is absorbed.

While the rice is boiling, heat the oil in a pan, add the fenugreek seeds and cook for a minute. Add the rest of the onion, the garlic, green chilli, ginger and the rest of the cumin, ground coriander and turmeric. Season and cook for 5 minutes on a low heat, stirring occasionally.

Add the spinach and cook for a further 15 minutes, stirring occasionally. Take off the heat.

In a frying pan heat a splash of oil and add the cubed marinated paneer. Cook until crisp on the outside, turning regularly.

Add the paneer to the spinach and mix in.

Finish with a sprinkling of the garam masala and chopped coriander.

Serve hot with poppadoms.

Monk Fish with Ginger and Lime

Serves 4

700g monk fish

juice of 2 limes

4 cloves garlic, finely chopped

4cm ginger

olive oil

salt and pepper

Chop the monk fish into 3cm cubes.

Place in a bowl large enough to be able to mix the fish with the other ingredients easily.

Add the lime juice and the garlic.

Using a swivel peeler slice the ginger into the bowl. Add enough olive oil to coat the fish (approximately 5 tbs) and season with pepper and a little salt.

Cover and leave in the fridge for at least 2 hours.

This works very well for a barbecue, in which case remove the monk fish from the marinade and cook for just a few minutes on each side until the fish is cooked through. Otherwise just fry in a little olive oil or grill.

Serve with white haricot beans – tinned, drained and rinsed will do fine. These can be dressed with lemon, olive oil, garlic and parsley, pepper and a little salt and roast tomatoes or a green salad.

Appendix A The Diagnosis and Management of Food Intolerance

According to conventional wisdom, before food is absorbed from the gut into the bloodstream it is first broken down into its smallest basic constituents. However, there is growing awareness that as a result of impaired digestion and/or 'leakiness' in the gut wall, incompletely digested food can make its way into the body where it can trigger unwanted reactions. Such reactions, often termed 'food sensitivity' or 'food intolerance', can cause a range of symptoms including fatigue, mental fogginess, irritable bowel syndrome, eczema, asthma and headaches. For those with a food-intolerance issue, its diagnosis and management may have significant benefits for health and well-being.

The Difference between Food 'Allergy' and 'Intolerance'

Many of us will be familiar with the life-threatening reaction some individuals suffer after eating peanuts, or the red rash that some will experience after eating strawberries. These sorts of reaction come on rapidly after eating a food, and are termed food 'allergy'. However, not all food reactions develop quickly, or are caused by the same mechanism that causes food allergy.

In many cases of food sensitivity, reactions can be delayed and can involve one or more mechanisms which may be difficult to identify. Such reactions, often collectively referred to as food 'intolerance', are the type of food reactions that concern us here.

The Physiology and Function of the Gut

To understand how food intolerance occurs, we first need to understand the process of digestion.

The role of digestion is to break food down into pieces small enough to pass through the gut wall and into the bloodstream. The fundamental processes in digestion are the action of chewing in the mouth, followed by the chemical breakdown of food by acid in the stomach and digestive enzymes and bile in the small intestine. In an ideal world, the body will digest food down into its smallest molecular constituents. Basically, this means starch, protein and fat being broken down into sugar, amino acids and so-called 'fatty acids' respectively.

However, should food not be completely digested, it has the capacity to 'leak' into the gut wall or through the gut wall into the bloodstream. Once this happens, the body may recognize these incompletely digested foods as 'foreign'. As a result, the body may react to these foods by mobilizing the immune or some other defence system. These reactions may be designed to neutralize a foreign food, but may also provoke one or more of a wide range of conditions and symptoms.

What Are the Symptoms of Food Intolerance?

Some of the conditions and symptoms of food intolerance include:

- Irritable bowel syndrome

- Abdominal bloating

- Lethargy, particularly within an hour or two of eating

- Mental 'fogginess' and low mood

- Childhood problems such as colic, glue ear, ear infections and recurrent tonsillitis

- Asthma

- Eczema

- Mucus or catarrh in the throat, nose or sinuses

- Fluid retention

- Inflammatory bowel disease such as Crohn's disease

- Headaches and migraine

What Causes Food Intolerance?

In healthy people, food reactions can be prevented by a healthy gut wall, which prevents entry of partially digested food. However, many factors are known to be able to cause 'leakiness' in the gut. These include alcohol, prescription medication (especially non-steroidal anti-inflammatory drugs), imbalance in the organisms in the gut (see Appendix B for more details about this) and nutritional deficiencies.

Another common underlying factor in food intolerance is inadequate digestion of food. This may be related to a general problem with digestion – something that we shall be covering in more depth later on in this Appendix. However, poor digestion may also relate to the fact that a food is simply not that easy to digest. Two substances that seem to have particular relevance here are the proteins 'casein' (found in dairy products) and 'gluten' (found in grains such as wheat, oats, rye and barley). For more details about why these foods are such common causes of food intolerance, see Chapters 4 (Against the Grain) and 6 (Slaying the Sacred Cow).

Testing for Food Intolerance

Food sensitivities can be tested for in a variety of ways. All have pros and cons.

Scratch Testing and IgE Blood Testing

The scratch test, also known as the prick test or patch test, involves breaching the outer layer of the skin, after which an extract of the food being tested is applied to the skin. Redness and swelling at the site of the test indicates a sensitivity to whatever is being tested. Another form of testing involves detection of what are known as IgE antibodies to specific foods in the blood.

These tests are quite useful for identifying 'allergic' reactions that tend to occur quickly after the ingestion of a food, but are generally ineffective for the diagnosis of the sorts of food sensitivity that concern us here.

IgG Blood Testing

Food intolerance can be due to immune reactions that involve the production of an antibody known as IgG, as distinct from the IgE antibodies that cause food allergy. Blood tests are available that detect the levels of this particular form of antibody to specific foods.

The Cytotoxic/ALCAT Test

Another way of assessing food-sensitivity reactions is to mix food extracts with immune cells, to find out which foods (if any) cause the immune cells to react. The cytotoxic and ALCAT blood tests make use of this method to diagnose food intolerance.

Electrodermal Testing

Electrodermal testing involves measuring the electrical current that flows through an acupuncture point, and then detecting any changes in this as the body is 'challenged' with individual foods. Changes in the electrical current flow through the acupuncture point as a food is tested suggest that there is a problem with this food. In skilled hands, this method can give good results, which are instantaneous.

Applied Kinesiology

This is similar to electrodermal testing, except that the practitioner measures muscle strength in response to foods rather than via an electrical current flowing through the body. Typically, muscle strength is first ascertained by the practitioner pressing down on the subject's outstretched arm. This is repeated while challenging the subject with foods, either by having them close to or in contact with the body, or by putting samples of food under the tongue. Like electrodermal testing, I've found the results obtained via this form of testing to be relatively reliable in skilled hands, and the results are immediate. This type of testing tends to be inexpensive compared to blood tests for food intolerance.

Which Tests Are Best?

While blood-testing for food intolerance has merit, I personally generally prefer methods such as electrodermal testing and kinesiology. These tests sometimes have an image of subjectivity and unreliability. Certainly these can be issues, but it needs to be borne in mind that the reliability of blood tests is far from assured. The main reason that I favour electrodermal testing and kinesiology is that they seem to pick up intolerances, whatever their precise mechanism. This is in distinct contrast to blood tests, each of which focuses on one *specific* type of reaction in the body. That's fine if your problems are due to the particular type of reaction being tested, but what if they're not? Basically, just because a food appears not to be a problem on a specific blood test does not mean there isn't a problem with that food at all. Because electrodermal testing and kinesiology take a broader sweep, my experience is that food sensitivities are less likely to be missed.

However, these techniques do depend, to some degree, on the skill and experience of the practitioner using them. There is no simple solution to this. However, you may want to enquire about the experience of any practitioner you are planning to see.

DIY Testing – the Elimination Diet

The elimination diet is regarded by many practitioners of nutritional medicine as the most accurate way of testing for food intolerance. The concept is simple: all likely problem foods are removed from the diet for a period of time. Once the symptoms or conditions being treated are alleviated, foods can be added back into the diet, one at a time, and a note is made of those foods which cause a recurrence of the symptoms.

Knowing which foods to eliminate from the diet is an art in itself. To help you, here is some guidance:

- Eliminate all sources of wheat (a very common problem food) from the diet. This includes most breads, pasta, pastry, pizza, biscuits, cakes, wheat-based breakfast cereals, wheat crackers, breaded food, battered food and anything containing flour.

- Eliminate milk, cheese and yoghurt from the diet (common problem foods, especially milk and cheese).

- Eliminate foods and drinks which you consume repeatedly, say on four or more days each week (the more of a food you eat, the more likely it is to be a problem).

- Eliminate the foods and drinks which you crave and think you might not be able to do without (it's not uncommon for individuals to 'crave' the foods they are sensitive to).

- Eliminate the foods and drinks which you suspect you may be reacting to.

You may wish to refer to the recipes in this book, most of which have been constructed to avoid the common culprit foods.

If you do indeed suffer from food intolerance and have eliminated your problem foods, you may well be feeling much better after a week or two on this regime. If this is the case, then it's time to start re-testing foods.

Take one of the foods you have eliminated and have a substantial portion of it one morning. A glass of milk at breakfast is an example. Over the next few hours, keep a look out for any symptoms that suggest food intolerance. These include a return of your original symptoms, with or without other symptoms including headache, low mood, fatigue and foggy thinking. If you get any reaction, make a note that the provoking food is one of your sensitivities, and eliminate it again from your diet. If you get no reaction to your first exposure to the food, try it again at lunch and dinner. If by the following morning you are totally free from symptoms, add it – provisionally – to a list of 'safe' foods.

For the next three days, re-eliminate the food and keep a watchful eye out for any symptoms that suggest a food reaction. It is possible that the symptoms of a reaction can come on two or three days after a food or drink is consumed. If such a reaction occurs, then you should suspect this food. If you still feel well after the three-day break, you can be pretty sure the foodstuff you are testing is fine for you.

In this way, proceed through the major foods you have eliminated, making a note of safe and unsafe foods as you go.

Overcoming Food Sensitivities in the Long Term

The first step in overcoming food sensitivities is to avoid the problem foods. In normal circumstances it is wise for problem foods to be excluded from the diet for a month. Two months is generally better if you can manage it. Many individuals find that after two months of exclusion of a food, they can go back to eating it without suffering the adverse effects they experienced before. However, with regard to food reintroduction, there are few things that need to be borne in mind:

1. **For some time after a food is excluded from the diet, the body's reaction to it is often worse than it was before.**
   Even though exclusion of a food from the diet is ultimately likely to lead to greater tolerance to that food, it can take a month or two or longer for this to occur. In fact, for some time after the point of exclusion it is common for an adverse reaction to a food to be worse than it was before.

2. When a food is reintroduced, it is best not to eat too much of it, too frequently.

It is usually possible to reintroduce a problem food back into the diet, and not have problems with it. However, if that food is eaten in relatively large quantities and/or is eaten quite frequently, then this increases the risk of the original problems recurring. For instance, if you find that you have an intolerance to wheat, excluding it for a couple of months and then returning to a wheat-based cereal in the morning and a sandwich for lunch will almost certainly trigger a recurrence of your original symptoms. However, confining yourself to the occasional bowl of pasta or sandwich may be fine.

3. In the long term, food sensitivities can be reduced by improving digestion and healing the lining of the gut.

Earlier in this Appendix we have discussed how poor digestion and leakiness in the intestinal wall can be at the root of a food-intolerance problem. Combating these issues can reduce the likelihood of old sensitivities returning or new ones developing.

Improving Digestion

While many of us take efficient and complete digestion of food for granted, my experience is that many of us are not particularly good digesters of food. Symptoms suggestive of this include indigestion, acid reflux and burping after meals. Some individuals feel they get full quickly, or find that food, especially a large meal, can get 'stuck' a bit. Bloating high up in the abdomen quite soon after a meal is another symptom that suggests poor digestion.

Simple approaches that can help to enhance digestion include:

Chew Your Food Thoroughly

Proper chewing is essential for proper digestion. Chewing stimulates the secretion of acid and digestive enzymes. Chewing also mixes food with saliva, which contains an enzyme which itself starts the digestion of starchy foods such as bread, potatoes, rice and pasta. And, perhaps most importantly of all, chewing breaks food up, massively increasing the surface area available for contact with the digestive juices. This increases the efficiency of digestion by giving stomach acid and digestive enzymes the opportunity to penetrate the food and do the digestive work. Each mouthful should ideally be chewed to a cream before swallowing.

Avoid Big Meals

The larger the meal, the larger the load on the digestive system. Small, frequent meals ease the burden on the digestive system and reduce the risk of incomplete digestion.

Avoid Drinking with Meals

Some people tend to drink quite a lot of fluid with meals, and believe that this can only help to 'wash food down'. The reality is quite the reverse. Drinking with meals dilutes the acid and enzymes that do the digestive work, and does nothing to help the process of digestion. In the main part, drinking should be done between meals, not at meal time.

Consider Food Combining

Foods are made up of several chemical constituents including protein, carbohydrate, fat, vitamins, minerals, fibre and water. The common protein-rich foods include meat, fish, dairy products and eggs. Common carbohydrates in the diet include bread, rice, pasta, breakfast cereals and potatoes. Proteins and carbohydrates are very different chemically, and are digested by different enzymes in the gut. In addition, proteins are initially digested in acid, while carbohydrates are better digested in alkali (quite the opposite).

While conventional wisdom dictates that the gut should be able to digest a mishmash of food perfectly well, gut physiology dictates that mixing protein and starch at meals tends to make harder digestive work than having just one of these foods at a time. The core principle of 'food combining' is to avoid the eating of protein-based foods with carbohydrate-dense foods at meals. According to this principle, meals consisting of meat or fish with salad or vegetables (other than the potato) are permissible, as are vegetable curry and rice or pasta with a red sauce and salad.

In theory at least, such meals should be more easily, quickly and completely digested than protein/starch combinations. One benefit of better digestion is that it helps the body extract more nutritional value from the food we eat. Complete digestion of food also reduces the potential for food sensitivity.

While I do not believe that food combining need be flawlessly adhered to by everyone, there are particular circumstances when it can be particularly useful. I generally recommend that individuals think about applying its principles in the evening, when digestive capacity can be at a bit of a low point. Also, my experience is that food combining almost always offers very significant relief to individuals suffering from indigestion and/or heartburn.

Supplementary Support for Individuals with Poor Digestion

Digestive capacity can be improved through the supplementation with capsules of acid and/or digestive enzymes. Generally speaking, digestive enzyme supplements can be used quite safely, and are normally taken after meals. However, acid supplements need to be handled with more care. They are best used in conjunction with advice from a suitably experienced practitioner.

For more information on supplements designed to assist digestion, see www.thetrueyoudiet.com.

Leakiness in the Gut Wall

Tests for leaky gut, known as tests for 'intestinal permeability' in the trade, are available via specialist laboratories. In this test, the subject drinks a fluid containing molecules of a range of sizes. The urine is then collected and analysed for these molecules. If large molecules are found in the urine, this suggests leakiness in the gut.

Supplementary Support for Gut Leakiness

Certain nutrients have an important role to play in healing the gut lining. Some of the important nutrients in this respect include glutamine and N-acetyl glucosamine (NAG).

For more information on supplements designed to heal leaky gut, see www.thetrueyoudiet.com.

Appendix B The Diagnosis and Management of Candida and Gut Dysbiosis

Within the gut reside large numbers of 'healthy' bacteria. These play an important role in several body processes including digestion, protection from unhealthy organisms, and the health and integrity of the gut lining. In certain circumstances, this internal 'ecosystem' can become imbalanced. Here, healthy bacteria can be lost and/or there can be overgrowth of potentially unhealthy organisms. This imbalance is often referred to as 'gut dysbiosis'.

One very common feature in gut dysbiosis is an overgrowth of the yeast organism 'Candida'. This issue can provoke symptoms such as bloating, wind, an irregular bowel habit and irritable bowel syndrome, fatigue and mental fogginess. For affected individuals, the identification and management of gut dysbiosis may have significant benefits for health and well-being.

The Physiology and Function of the Internal Ecosystem

The gut is by no means a sterile environment. Each of us holds about 1½ to 2kg of bacteria in our intestinal tracts. The gut can also contain potentially unhealthy organisms such as yeast and parasites. In health, even if such organisms exist in the gut, a preponderance of healthy bacteria will generally maintain normal gut function. Not uncommonly, though, certain factors can disrupt the balance of organisms in the gut. One quite frequent particular issue here is overgrowth in a yeast (fungal) species known as 'Candida'.

What Are the Symptoms of Candida?

Candida overgrowth can cause a range of symptoms which include:

*   **Abdominal bloating and/or wind**
    Yeast is a 'fermenting' organism, which means it can produce gas that may manifest as abdominal bloating and/or wind.

- **Altered bowel habit**

  For many individuals with Candida, bowel habit can be somewhat erratic. Not uncommonly there can be a tendency for the bowel habit to alternate between constipation and loose bowel motions.

- **Unexplained fatigue and/or mental 'fogginess'**

- **Anal itching**

- **Vaginal yeast infection (thrush)**

- **Fungal skin infections including athlete's foot and itching/rash in the groin**

What Causes Candida Overgrowth?

One reason why overgrowth of this organism seems so common relates to the use of antibiotics. While these are designed to kill harmful bacteria in the body, antibiotics also have enormous potential to cut a swathe through the healthy gut bacteria. However, because they do not kill yeast, this can lead to an overgrowth of yeast species. Other factors that may encourage yeast growth include a diet rich in yeast-encouraging foods (such as sugar, refined starches, soy sauce, beer, wine and bread), stress, and taking the oral contraceptive pill.

Testing for Candida

Candida can be tested for using a variety of means including stool tests (these may identify the presence of actual yeast organisms) or blood tests (which identify antibodies to either the yeast or to the part of the yeast that the body reacts to, known as the 'antigen').

Another test for yeast is known as the 'gut fermentation test'. In this test a blood sample is taken and then the individual being tested is given a measured dose of sugar. An hour later, another sample of blood is taken. Both blood samples are analysed for various fermentation products including alcohol. The presence of these substances in significant quantities can point to the presence of excess yeast in the gut.

It is possible to diagnose yeast overgrowth through a number of non-laboratory tests including electrodermal testing and applied kinesiology. These forms of testing have their own merits, especially if carried out by an experienced and skilled practitioner. Assessment is usually relatively cheap and the results are immediate. Another advantage with these forms of testing is that they can allow contact with a practitioner who may be able to guide you through the intricacies of an anti-Candida programme, should testing show this to be a problem.

The Anti-Candida Diet

The cornerstone of the anti-Candida approach is a diet which helps starve yeast out of the system. This means an avoidance of foods which feed yeast directly or encourage yeast by being yeasty, mouldy or fermented in their own right.

Yeast-feeding Foods to Avoid

* Sugar

* Sweetening agents such as maple syrup, molasses, honey and malt syrup

* Sugar-containing foods such as biscuits, cakes, confectionery, ice cream, pastries, sugared breakfast cereals, soft drinks and fruit juice

* White flour products including white bread, crackers, pizza and pasta

Yeasty, Mouldy or Fermented Foods to Avoid

* Bread and other yeast-raised items

* Alcoholic drinks, particularly beer and wine which are very yeasty

* Gravy mixes (most contain brewer's yeast)

* Vinegar and vinegar-containing foods such as ketchup (which also contains sugar), mustard, mayonnaise and many prepared salad dressings

* Pickles, miso, tempeh and soy sauce (all fermented)

* Aged cheeses including Cheddar, Stilton, Swiss, Brie and Camembert (cheese is inherently mouldy)

* Peanuts (and peanut butter) and pistachios (these foods tend to harbour yeast)

* Mushrooms

- Dried fruit (these are intensely sugary and tend to harbour mould)

- Yeast-containing foods such as soups and pre-packaged foods

Foods to Eat Freely
The foods which are generally very safe to eat on an anti-Candida regime are listed below.

Protein-rich Foods
- Eggs

- Fish including naturally smoked fish

- Shellfish

- Chicken

- Turkey

- Lamb

- Beef

- Pork

- Duck

- Tofu (soya bean curd)

- Lettuce

- Tomato

- Cucumber

- Celery

- Cabbage

- Broccoli

- Cauliflower

- Spinach

- Chard

- Kale

- Watercress

- Brussels sprouts

- Asparagus

- Onion

- Leek

- Green beans

- Parsnips

- Aubergine

- Artichoke

- Avocado

Foods to Be Eaten in Moderation

Certain foods such as grains, high-starch vegetables, legumes or pulses can be eaten on an anti-Candida regime. However, it's best not to eat masses of them because they do tend to have some fermentation potential. The bulk of the diet should be based around the foods which can be eaten freely, supplemented with more limited amounts of:

High-starch Vegetables
- Potatoes

- Sweet potatoes

- Squash (e.g. butternut)

Beans and lentils

Grains
- Yeast-free rye bread

- Rye crackers

- Brown rice

- Wild rice

- Brown rice cakes

- Barley

- Millet

- Oats, oat cakes and oat-based breakfast cereals

- Buckwheat

- Quinoa

- Spelt wheat

Fruit

Whether or not fruit is advisable on an anti-Candida regime is a real moot point. Some practitioners say it can be eaten freely, others say it should be completely excluded, at least to begin with. My experience is that one or two pieces of fruit a day is generally very well tolerated, though I would avoid grapes, which are intensely sugary and usually are covered in a mouldy bloom. All fruit that you're not going to peel prior to eating should be washed thoroughly. The best fruits are berries, as these contain the least sugar. Dried fruits, as mentioned before, are not advisable on an anti-Candida diet.

Menu Suggestions

The principles of the anti-Candida diet have been incorporated in the recipes to be found in this book. One exception here is the dried fruit to be found in the muesli recipe. This should be omitted by those on an anti-Candida diet.

Supplementary Support for Candida
Probiotics

Probiotics are supplements of healthy gut bacteria. These supplements, ideally, should contain a range of organisms. Also, making good probiotic supplements is not easy, as the organisms can perish during their production, or perhaps not survive the harsh acidic environment in the stomach. For more information on suitable probiotic supplements, see www.thetrueyoudiet.com.

Anti-fungal Supplements

There are some natural agents that may be useful in combating yeast in the body.

Oregano

Oregano has been employed as an antiseptic in herbal and folk medicine for thousands of years. Oregano contains a number of active ingredients; probably the two most important of which are carvacrol and thymol. Studies have shown that oregano has anti-fungal properties and can inhibit the growth of Candida.

Garlic

Like oregano, garlic has a tradition of use in herbal medicine that goes back thousands of years. Garlic has the ability to kill a range of organisms including bacteria, viruses, parasites and fungi. In natural medicine garlic is a widely used substance in the control and eradication of Candida.

Grapefruit Seed Extract

Extracts of grapefruit seed are thought to have the ability to kill Candida in the body. Many Candida sufferers report that taking grapefruit seed extract has helped them control their symptoms and conquer their yeast-related problems.

For more information on natural anti-fungal supplements, see www.thetrueyoudiet.com.

Parasites and Gut Dysbiosis

Candida is a common organism found in gut dysbiosis, but it's not the only one. A reasonably common cause of persistent dysbiosis is parasites such as 'Blastocystis hominis' and 'Dientamoeba fragilis'. Sometimes, specialized testing and treatment are required for parasitic infection. See www.thetrueyoudiet.com for details.

Appendix C The Diagnosis and Management of Adrenal Weakness

The body has two adrenal glands, which sit on top of the kidneys. These glands play a role in many body processes including the regulation of blood-sugar levels and immune function. The adrenal glands have a particularly important part to play in our body's response to stress. In fact, these organs are chiefly responsible for orchestrating changes in the body that allow us to cope with and adapt to whatever physical and emotional challenges we face in our lives.

In some individuals, the function of the adrenal glands can become 'weakened'. In the long term this may lead to symptoms such as fatigue, low mood, susceptibility to infection and allergies, low blood pressure or cravings for sugar and/or salt. For some individuals, weakened adrenal function can cause long-term health issues that can be very debilitating, including chronic fatigue syndrome. This Appendix examines the common features of adrenal weakness, and how this condition may be diagnosed and managed.

While anyone may suffer from adrenal weakness, my experience is that it is more common in individuals of the 'hunter' type.

The Physiology and Function of the Adrenal Glands
The function of the adrenal glands is to produce hormones that have a critical role to play in many processes, including the body's response to stress. Let's take a look at some of the hormones produced by the adrenal glands.

Adrenaline
Adrenaline is one of the main hormones secreted by the adrenal glands in the stress response. Among other things, adrenaline increases the heart

rate and blood pressure. The action of adrenaline also increases blood-sugar levels by stimulating the conversion of glycogen (a starch-like substance stored in the liver and muscles) into glucose. Adrenaline has a relatively short duration of action in the body.

Cortisol

The other main stress hormone secreted by the adrenal glands is cortisol. However, while adrenaline has a relatively short duration of action in the body, cortisol's actions in the body tend to linger more. Like adrenaline, cortisol tends to increase blood-sugar levels, partly through its ability to stimulate the conversion of non-carbohydrate fuels such as amino acids (the building-blocks of protein) into glucose.

Cortisol also has very important roles in the regulation of various body systems including the immune system and the control of inflammation in the body. Prolonged stress can cause higher-than-normal levels of cortisol which may in turn lead to problems such as impairment of the immune system, loss of muscle mass, bone loss, insomnia and depression.

Dihydroepiandrosterone (DHEA)

DHEA is actually the most plentiful hormone secreted by the adrenal glands. It has a number of regulating roles in the body, including helping in the growth and repair of proteins in body tissues, especially muscle. This hormone also plays a part in the processes that heal tissues after injury or infection. In addition, DHEA can be converted into other hormones, principally testosterone and oestrogen, which themselves have important actions within the body.

Aldosterone

Aldosterone participates in the regulation of minerals in the body. Specifically, it preserves sodium in the body, whilst at the same time encouraging the loss of potassium. These actions help to maintain fluid levels and blood pressure

Adrenal Weakness

In some individuals, adrenal function may be somewhat weakened. This condition is sometimes referred to as 'hypoadrenalism', 'adrenal exhaustion' or 'adrenal weakness'. It is important to distinguish this state from a condition known as Addison's disease (also known as 'adrenal insufficiency') in which there is extreme failure of adrenal function. For more about this distinction, see the section on conventional medical testing below.

What Are the Symptoms of Adrenal Weakness?
Some of the most prominent symptoms of adrenal weakness include:

Fatigue
Adrenally weakened individuals tend to be tired. They often lack the vitality they once took for granted. They quite often have to force themselves through the day, and may prop themselves up with caffeine to give them the energy they need to complete whatever tasks they face. As time goes on these individuals often feel the need to take more sleep. However, it is not uncommon for an adrenally compromised person to feel very tired on waking, irrespective of how much sleep they get.

Easy Fatigue and Lack of Resilience
Adrenally weakened individuals often have little in the way of energy 'reserve'. Not only do they generally feel tired, but they often get tired out or exhausted quite easily. For individuals with adrenal compromise, any additional stress on the body, be it of a physiological and/or emotional nature, causes real energy lows. A busy week at work, the stress associated with a child's illness, or a couple of late nights can be all it takes to bring energy crashing down.

One activity that tends to bring this to the fore is exercise. Individuals with good adrenal function tend to feel buoyed up and energized by exercise. While adrenally weakened individuals may feel *emotionally* satis fied to have taken exercise, the fact is it can lead them to feel physically tired and 'wiped out' the same day or the day after.

Insomnia
Adrenally compromised individuals can often get a 'boost' of energy in the mid–late evening which can cause them to have difficulty getting off to sleep. Also, they can be prone to dropping their blood-sugar level in the night, which essentially turns on the body's stress response. This can cause waking in the night, typically at 3.30–4.30 a.m. Individuals can find themselves quite alert at this time, and may find that they are unable to get back to sleep again until, often, about half an hour before the alarm goes off.

Low Blood Pressure

Stress is often thought to cause raised blood pressure. However, long-term stress, through its effects on adrenal function, can actually lead to *low* blood pressure (hypotension) in time. Adrenally weakened individuals often have a blood pressure of 110/70 mmHg or less. These individuals also tend to have a blood pressure which drops on standing from a seated or lying position. This condition, the medical term for which is 'postural hypotension', can cause dizziness on standing.

Salt Craving

Some individuals with adrenal weakness will crave salt. It is thought that what might be going on here is that the body is demanding more salt to help replenish sodium, which is not being retained due to a lack of aldosterone and/or other hormones.

Sugar Craving

Adrenally compromised individuals can often crave sugary foods such as biscuits or chocolate. This is usually a sign of the episodes of low blood sugar they are prone to.

The Need to Eat Regularly

Individuals with adrenal weakness tend to need to eat regularly to keep them from feeling weak, light-headed or 'shaky'. If the body is not being fuelled from the outside (by eating), the body needs to generate sugar from the breakdown of stored fuels in the body, such as glycogen in the liver. If the adrenal glands are weakened it is possible that the stress hormones such as cortisol are not made in sufficient quantities to enable adequate amounts of sugar to be mobilized in this way.

An Increased Tendency to Allergic Conditions

One other symptom suffered by adrenally weakened individuals is an increased tendency to allergic conditions such as hay fever and asthma.

What Causes the Adrenal Glands to Weaken?

It is likely that, through the process of evolution, our adrenal glands became adapted to coping with relatively short and defined periods of stress. However, these days, the frenetic pace of life and the challenges brought by modern-day living can cause the adrenal glands to weaken in time. Almost incessant stimulation of the adrenal glands can take its toll eventually.

In my experience, adrenal weakness almost always manifests in individuals who are 'doers'. Usually from an early age, these individuals have been used to packing a lot into the day. As children these individuals are often quite academic and competitive, possibly with a sporty bent. They often progress to busy jobs with long working hours. If they are women and have opted for a family, usually they are juggling a number of different commitments. Some individuals describe themselves as chronically 'stressed', and are often consumed with personal, financial and/or work-related pressures.

Many individuals find that their adrenal weakness comes on relatively suddenly. For instance, individuals can have very high levels of function and output for years, even decades. Then, perhaps over just a few weeks, they can seem to go into quite rapid decline after a period of particular stress or perhaps a viral infection or other illness.

A useful analogy is to think of the adrenal glands as a bit like a bank account, where the money in the account represents your energy. Imagine starting life out with, say, a million pounds in your account. Now imagine spending £100 per day in energy, but only making up £50 per day in 'interest' (through rest and recuperation). With a million in the bank to start with, it is possible to go for a very long time spending in this way with little or no sign of trouble. However, after several decades you would be 'in the red'. While you may have been used to spending a certain sum for many years, eventually your energy 'bank' starts to decline any further withdrawals. This helps explain why individuals used to a certain level of output can 'all of a sudden' find themselves unable to sustain the sort of lifestyle they may have had for years or even decades.

Conventional Laboratory Tests for Adrenal Function

To understand the laboratory tests for adrenal function, we first need to know about how adrenal function is regulated within the body. The secretion of stress hormones is governed by another hormone known as adrenocorticotrophic hormone (ACTH), which itself is produced by a small organ at the base of the brain known as the 'pituitary gland'. When we become stressed, the pituitary gland makes more ACTH, which stimulates the adrenal glands to make stress hormones such as cortisol. When the stress goes away, ACTH levels, in normal circumstances, decline and so does the production of stress hormones from the adrenal glands.

The main conventional medical test used is something called the 'short ACTH stimulation test' – also known as the 'Synacthen™' test. Here a blood sample is taken, after which an injection of ACTH is given. Half an hour later a second sample of blood is taken. The cortisol levels are measured in both samples. If the first sample shows a low level of cortisol, and/or if there is not a sufficient rise in the cortisol level in response to ACTH, further testing is usually advised.

Many doctors do not believe in the concept of adrenal weakness. The attitude here is usually that if blood tests do not show Addison's disease, then there is nothing wrong with adrenal-gland function. However, the 'normal' ranges for adrenal function are set very wide, and to be diagnosed with Addison's disease adrenal function needs to be very low indeed. It is possible, therefore, for someone to have very compromised adrenal function, but not so bad that Addison's disease is diagnosed. These individuals may nonetheless suffer from significant symptoms as a result of their suboptimal adrenal function.

Alternative Tests for Adrenal Function

Adrenal hormones can also be measured using saliva samples. One of the most commonly used tests is known as the adrenal stress index (ASI) test. Here, four saliva samples taken at intervals during the day are analysed for cortisol. Some tests measure DHEA at these four points too, while others measure DHEA at just one point in the day.

This test can be quite useful for assessing adrenal function because it allows assessment of how cortisol (and perhaps DHEA) levels change over the course of a day. This is generally more useful than taking a single reading of cortisol and/or DHEA.

My experience in practice is that individuals with quite significant adrenal weakness have relatively normal levels of cortisol, but low or low-normal levels of DHEA. In very severe adrenal weakness, levels of both cortisol and DHEA can be low.

My advice for individuals who feel they would like to have their adrenal function tested is to work with a practitioner who has experience in this area. More details about salivary hormone testing can be found at www.thetrueyoudiet.com.

Restoring Adrenal Health

The function of even quite compromised adrenal glands can usually be restored in time. The fundamental approach here is to take steps to build up the 'cash reserve' in our adrenal bank account. This basically means doing less that draws on our adrenal reserve, as well as doing more that helps 'interest' build up.

What this means for an individual will depend on the precise factors that are specific to that individual. However, common lifestyle adjustments that play a potential part in adrenal restoration include avoiding strenuous exercise, getting more sleep, reducing working hours and dealing with underlying emotional stresses. Nutritionally, it is very important to eat a diet that will give maximal support to the body. Fundamental to this is eating a diet appropriate for one's 'type'. In my experience, 'hunters' are more prone to adrenal weakness than other types. I find generally that these individuals will not feel well unless they eat a diet that is relatively rich in protein and fat.

Nutrients that Support the Adrenal Glands
Several nutrients seem to have particular ability to support adrenal gland function.

Vitamin C
The adrenal glands contain a higher concentration of vitamin C than anywhere else in the body, and this nutrient is believed to be important for the function of these organs. A good dose would be 0.5–1g of vitamin C, twice a day.

Vitamin B₅
Vitamin B_5, also known as pantothenic acid, is believed to be important for adrenal gland function. A good dose would be 500 mg, twice a day.

Ginseng
One of the most popular agents for treating adrenal weakness is ginseng. This comes in two main forms: Panax ginseng (also known as Korean ginseng) and Siberian ginseng.

Panax Ginseng
Panax ginseng is thought to be an adrenal 'tonic'. The normal dose is 100–200mg of standardized extract containing 4–7 per cent ginsenosides per day. The dose for non-standardized preparations is 1–2g per day or 2–3ml of herbal tincture. It is generally recommended that Panax ginseng

be used on a cyclical basis with treatment periods of two to three weeks interspersed with supplement-free periods of one to two weeks. While Panax ginseng is generally regarded as safe at the recommended dosage, it may cause insomnia if taken close to bedtime. It should not be used by those suffering from high blood pressure. Panax ginseng is known to cause breast tenderness and menstrual abnormalities in some women, and is not recommended for pregnant or lactating women.

Siberian Ginseng
The active ingredients in Siberian ginseng are thought to support the function of the adrenal glands. Siberian ginseng has been shown to sharpen the mind as well as improve physical energy. The recommended dose is 300–400mg of concentrated solid standardized extract each day. The normal dosage for dried powder is 2–3g per day. It is generally recommended that Siberian ginseng be used on a cyclical basis with treatment periods of six to eight weeks interspersed with breaks lasting one to two weeks.

Siberian ginseng may cause mild, transient diarrhoea and insomnia if taken too close to bedtime. Again, as with Panax ginseng, it should not be used by those suffering from high blood pressure. Siberian ginseng is not recommended for pregnant or lactating women.

Liquorice
Liquorice is a natural substance containing a compound called 'glycyrrhizin'. In the body, glycyrrhizin breaks down to glycyrrhetinic acid. Glycyrrhetinic acid has anti-inflammatory actions in the body, and also slows down the breakdown of cortisol. In this way, liquorice can enhance the effects of cortisol, and may help to 'take the strain off' the adrenal glands.

The normal recommended dose is 5–6g of whole liquorice root taken in two or three divided doses during the day. Alternatively, 250–500mg of concentrated extract can be taken three times a day.

High-dose liquorice can lead to sodium accumulation and a loss of the mineral potassium in the body. These changes may increase blood pressure. Even though this may have positive benefit for someone suffering from low blood pressure (hypotension), it does pose a small risk, too. For this reason it is best that liquorice be taken under the supervision of a practitioner experienced in its use.

Other herbs that may help support adrenal function include Withania ('Withania somnifera') and Rhodiola ('Sedum roseum').

For more information on supplements for supporting the adrenal glands, see www.thetrueyoudiet.com.

Hormone-based Supplements

In certain situations, especially where the level of one or more adrenal hormones is low, it may be beneficial to use hormone-based treatment to restore adrenal function and health.

Options here include cortisol and/or DHEA supplementation. Other possibilities are pregnenolone (from which both DHEA and cortisol can be made) and adrenal glandulars (supplements containing animal-derived adrenal gland tissues). I recommend working with a doctor experienced in the use of these agents.

Appendix D The Diagnosis and Management of Low Thyroid Function (Hypothyroidism)

The thyroid is a gland, about the size and shape of a bowtie, which sits in the front of the neck just above the top of the breastbone. The thyroid has a very big role to play in regulating the body's metabolism, which influences a diverse range of processes including body temperature, energy levels and the conversion of food into energy.

However, in some individuals thyroid function may be lower than normal, and this may cause a range of symptoms such as weight gain, fatigue, mental lethargy, depression, sensitivity to cold, and dry skin and hair. The diagnosis and management of low thyroid function can be vital in the attainment of optimal health and well-being.

While anyone may suffer from low thyroid function, my experience is that women are more commonly affected than men, particularly those of the 'gatherer' type.

The Physiology and Function of the Thyroid Gland

The thyroid produces a variety of hormones, the most plentiful of which is known as 'thyroxine' (also known as 'T4'). Outside the thyroid, T4 is converted into another hormone called 'tri-iodothyronine' (also known as 'T3'). T3 is actually a more active form of thyroid hormone. T3 basically stimulates cells to burn fuel with oxygen to release energy, some of this being released as heat. Essentially, the more T4 and T3 there is around, the faster the metabolism, the less tendency there is for weight gain and the warmer the body is.

The thyroid's production of hormones is itself regulated by a tiny gland located at the base of the brain known as the 'pituitary'. The pituitary, in turn, is regulated by a part of the brain known as the 'hypothalamus'. In health, if the hypothalamus senses a drop in the levels of T4 and/or T3, it sends a signal to the pituitary which in turn secretes a hormone known as 'thyroid-stimulating hormone' or 'TSH'. As its name suggests, this hormone instructs the thyroid to produce more thyroid hormones. In theory, as thyroid hormone levels rise, the hypothalamus instructs the pituitary to produce less TSH, which ensures thyroid hormone levels do not rise too high. This mechanism is designed to ensure stable levels of thyroid hormones in the body.

However, like any other gland or organ in the body, the thyroid gland can weaken. In this case, despite high levels of TSH it may still not be able to make the amounts of thyroid hormones necessary for optimal health. This low thyroid-function state is known as 'hypothyroidism'.

Most cases of hypothyroidism are due to a failure of the thyroid gland itself. However, it is possible for this condition to be the result of failure of the pituitary gland. Here, the pituitary fails to produce enough TSH to stimulate the thyroid sufficiently.

What Are the Symptoms of Hypothyroidism?
Weight Gain
Individuals can often gain weight for no obvious reason (e.g. quite sudden weight gain despite no change in exercise or dietary habits). They will often find it difficult to lose weight, too. For some, cutting back on their intake of food and/or stepping up their activity can lead to little or no weight loss.

Fatigue, Low Mood and/or Depression
Individuals with hypothyroidism are often consistently tired. They tend to feel 'slow and sluggish'. They can also be prone to low mental energy, which can manifest as low mood and depression.

Feet and Ankle Swelling
There is a tendency for individuals with hypothyroidism to retain salt, water and protein in the tissues. This can cause swelling, also known as 'oedema', which is often most noticeable in the feet and ankles.

Facial Changes
Individuals with hypothyroidism may experience puffiness of the eyelids, facial swelling and the loss or thinning of the outer portions of the eyebrows.

Enlarged Tongue

Hypothyroidism may cause enlargement of the tongue. As a result, the tongue may press against the inside of the lower teeth and its edge may appear 'scalloped'.

Dry Skin and Hair

Individuals with hypothyroidism often suffer from dry skin and/or hair.

Menstrual Symptoms

Women with hypothyroidism can suffer from heavy and/or irregular periods.

Infertility

Hypothyroidism is a quite common, but often undiagnosed, cause of infertility, especially in women.

What Causes Thyroid Weakness?

In theory, hypothyroidism can be caused by a range of factors including nutrient deficiency (particularly of iodine) and chemical pollutants. In my experience, one of the most potent underlying factors in this condition is *genetics*. I do find that a relatively high percentage of women with hypothyroidism have one or more female family members, such as a sister, mother, grandmother or aunt, with thyroid disease of some form.

Conventional Testing for Hypothyroidism

The conventional way to test thyroid function is to measure blood levels of thyroid-stimulating hormone (TSH). If this is raised, this suggests hypothyroidism. The diagnosis is usually confirmed by measuring T4 levels, which are characteristically low in cases of hypothyroidism.

While the TSH test is generally seen by doctors and endocrinologists as a sensitive and accurate guide to thyroid function, the reality is that this test has a number of deficiencies.

One major issue here relates to the 'normal range' set for TSH. Normal ranges are designed to encompass 95 per cent of people. What this means is that to have an elevated TSH, one needs to be in the top 2.5 per cent of the population for TSH levels. This means that however common hypothyroidism may be, only a relatively small proportion of the population can be diagnosed using this test.

Also, as discussed earlier, low thyroid function can be related to low pituitary function. In traditional medicine, lower-than-normal levels of TSH are believed to signify this. However, before the pituitary is exhausted to this extent it is possible for it to go through a phase where TSH levels are considered 'normal' even though thyroid function is significantly compromised. While this notion is plausible, it is generally not accepted by endocrinologists (doctors specializing in hormone-related disease).

Another problem with conventional testing is that it relies on levels of TSH and, usually, T4. If there is enough T4 in the body, the brain can sense this and feel there is no need to increase TSH production. However, T4 is not very active in the rest of the body – it seems T3 has a more important role to play in this respect. It is therefore possible for someone to have enough T4 but not enough T3, and be hypothyroid as a result. T3 levels are rarely checked in conventional medicine, meaning someone with low T3 levels – who is hypothyroid as a result – can get missed because 'normal' TSH and T4 levels are found.

Yet another potential deficiency of conventional thyroid testing is that while it may show the level of hormones in the bloodstream, it does not tell us how active and effective those hormones are. It is now well recognized, for instance, that individuals can become resistant to the hormone insulin (known as 'insulin resistance'), which may eventually lead to a problem with diabetes. In contrast, the concept of thyroid-hormone resistance has yet to catch on in conventional medical circles.

I believe that thyroid-function testing should be performed both in the establishment of the diagnosis and its management. However, I think there is a strong case for measuring T3 levels as well as those of TSH and T4. In addition, I believe that the test results need to be taken in the context of the clinical symptoms and signs an individual is exhibiting. In practice this means that treatment may be deemed appropriate for individuals who appear 'normal' on conventional testing.

The Barnes Test

The Barnes test uses body temperature on waking to assess thyroid function.

Start by taking a mercury thermometer, shaking it down and leaving it by your bed before you go to sleep. On waking, before getting up, place the bulb of the thermometer under your armpit and wait for a full 10 minutes. Record the temperature. Repeat this over a few days.

For women still having menstrual periods, this is best done on days 2, 3 and 4 of the period itself. Once you have at least three readings, work out the average. The normal body temperature in the morning is between 36.6 and 36.8°C (97.8–98.2°F). A temperature of 36.4°C (97.4°F) or less suggests low thyroid function.

Restoring Thyroid Health

Thyroid support can, broadly speaking, come in the form of diet, natural remedies and hormone-based therapies. From a nutritional perspective, eating according to one's 'type' is important. My experience is that the majority of hypothyroid individuals are 'gatherers'. In addition, it is important to bear in mind that certain foods contain compounds that can disrupt thyroid function. The principal foods to avoid are soy (in any form) and vegetables from the 'brassica' class such as broccoli, Brussels sprouts, cabbage, cauliflower and kale. These vegetables, also known as *cruciferous* vegetables, contain substances known as glucosinolates which can convert into substances that disrupt thyroid function. However, evidence suggests that the enzyme responsible for converting glucosinolates into thyroid-toxic compounds is deactivated during the cooking process[1] What this means is that brassica vegetables are likely to be suitable for individuals with hypothyroidism, as long as they are cooked first.

Natural Supplements for the Thyroid

There are several herbs and nutrients which may be of benefit in supporting thyroid function.

Iodine

Iodine is an essential component of the thyroid hormones, and without it the thyroid simply cannot make these hormones in sufficient quantity. Supplementing with iodine, for instance in the form of kelp or dulce, may therefore help to improve thyroid function.

Caution
High levels of iodine may in fact suppress thyroid function. Do not exceed 500mcg per day unless under the instruction of a doctor with expertise in this area.

Selenium

Selenium participates in the conversion of T4 into T3; a deficiency of selenium may stall this process. Other studies have also linked low levels of selenium with hypothyroidism.

Caution
Very high levels of selenium may actually lower levels of T3. It is important, therefore, not to exceed 300mcg per day unless under the advice of a doctor.

L-Tyrosine

L-Tyrosine is an amino acid (building-block of protein) which has an essential role in the formation of thyroid hormones. L-Tyrosine can help in the treatment of hypothyroidism.

For more information on supplements suitable for supporting the thyroid, see www.thetrueyoudiet.com.

Hormone-based Treatments for Hypothyroidism

The conventional medical approach to hypothyroidism is centred on the use of a synthetic version of the hormone thyroxine (T4). This is normally administered initially at a dose of 25–100mcg per day, and increased in doses of 25–50mcg every three or four weeks until TSH levels come into the normal range. The usual maintenance dose is between 100 and 200mcg per day.

Certainly, some hypothyroid individuals feel significant benefit from taking thyroxine in the right dose. However, there are also many others who do not. Often, individuals who have been diagnosed hypothyroid feel little or no better on thyroxine treatment.

One reason for this may be that some individuals may have a problem converting thyroxine to T3 – the active form of the hormone. If you are currently taking thyroxine and feel it is not doing as much for you as you would like, then it might be worthwhile having your T3 level checked. As discussed above, this hormone is not routinely tested in the UK and you may experience some resistance from your doctor should you request it. If your T3 level is found to be low or low-normal, then it might help to take selenium, because of this nutrient's ability to help the conversion of T4 to T3. I suggest 200–300mcg per day.

Some, though not many, doctors will prescribe T3 for hypothyroidism, usually in combination with T4. This obviously gets round any problem there may be with the conversion of thyroxine into T3. T3 has a much shorter duration of action in the body, and levels of this hormone can be harder to regularize than T4. However, for certain individuals T3 seems to help in a way that T4 on its own may not.

Thyroid Glandulars

Some doctors, usually naturally oriented ones, will treat hypothyroidism with what are known as 'thyroid glandulars'. As their name suggests, these contain thyroid gland tissue, usually obtained from pigs. It is believed that the range of hormones available in a glandular supplement is much more likely to have a beneficial effect on hypothyroid individuals than the single hormone (thyroxine) usually deployed in conventional treatment. Also, thyroid glandulars are believed to contain a hormone secreted by the thyroid known as di-iodotyrosine (also known as T2), which may have an important but as yet unrecognized role to play in healthy thyroid function.

Many individuals who do not do well on thyroxine seem to respond much better to glandular supplements. The most widely used thyroid glandular in the US is a product called 'Armour thyroid'. The dosing of Armour thyroid is in units known as 'grains'. One grain of Armour thyroid contains 38mcg of T4 and 9mcg of T3. In my experience, adults often require a maintenance dose of between one and three grains a day.

Cautions

I recommend that anyone considering using thyroid glandulars should work with a doctor with experience and expertise in this area. Thyroid glandulars must be used with special caution in individuals with a history of heart disease. Thyroid glandulars, if taken in excess, do have the potential for side-effects such as anxiety, nervousness, palpitations, excessive weight loss and insomnia. More details about the diagnosis and management of hypothyroidism can be had via the website www.thyroiduk.org. This site also holds a list of practitioners who take a holistic approach to thyroid treatment, many of whom use thyroid glandular products where these are considered appropriate.

References

Introduction

1. Yancy, W S Jr *et al.* 'A low-carbohydrate, ketogenic diet versus a low-fat diet to treat obesity and hyperlipidemia: a randomized, controlled trial', *Ann Intern Med* 2004; 18; 140(10): 769–77

Chapter 1

1. Boesch, C *et al.* 'Hunting behaviour of wild chimpanzees in the Tai national park', *Am J Phys Anthropol* 1989; 78: 547–73
2. Goodall, J 'Continuities between chimpanzee and human behaviour', in Isaac, G and McCown, E (eds), *Human Origins: Louis Leakey and the East African Evidence* (Menlo Park, CA: Benjamin, 1976)
3. Goodman, M *et al.* 'Molecular phylogeny of the family of apes and humans', *Genome* 1989; 31: 316–35
4. Brunet, M *et al.* 'A new hominid from the upper Miocene of Chad, central Africa', *Nature* 2002; 418: 145–51
5. Wrangham, R and Peterson, D *Demonic Males: Apes and the Origins of Human Violence* (London: Bloomsbury, 1996)
6. White, T D *et al.* 'Australopithecus ramidus, a new species of early hominid from Aramis, Ethiopia', *Nature* 1994; 371: 306–12
7. Wrangham and Peterson op cit
8. White T D *et al.* 'Jaws and teeth of Australopithecus afarensis from Maka, Middle Awash, Ethiopia', *Am J Phys Anthropol* 2000; 111: 45–68
9. Stanley, V 'Paleoecology of the Arctic-Steppe mammoth biome', *Curr Anthropol* 1980; 21: 663–6
10. Walker, A and Shipman, P *The Wisdom of the Bones: In Search of Human Origins* (New York: Alfred A. Knopf, 1996)
11. Rose, L *et al.* 'Meat eating, hominid sociality, and home bases revisited', *Curr Anthropol* 1996; 37: 307–38

12. Cordain L *et al.* 'Fatty acid composition and energy density of foods available to African hominids: evolutionary implications for human brain development', *Wld Rev Nutr Diet* 2001; 90: 144–61
13. Wrangham and Peterson op cit
14. Burenhult, G 'Towards homo sapiens: habilines, erectines, and neanderthals', in Burenhult, G (ed.), *The First Humans: Human Origins and History to 10,000 BC* (New York: HarperCollins, 1993)
15. Scarre, C (ed.) *Smithsonian Timelines of the Ancient World: A Visual Chronology from the Origins of Life to AD 1500* (New York: Dorling Kindersley, 1993)
16. Ambrose, S H 'Isotopic analysis of paleodiets: Methodological and interpretive considerations', in Sandford, M K (ed.), *Investigations of Ancient Human Tissue* (Chemical Analyses in Anthropology, 1993)
17. Langhorne, P A *et al.* 'Controlled diet and climate experiments on nitrogen isotope ratios of rats', in Ambrose, S H and Katzenburg, M A (eds), *Biogeochemical Approaches to Palaeodietary Analysis* (New York: Kluwer Academic/Plenum Press, 2000)
18. Ambrose, S H and Norr, L 'Experimental evidence for the relationship of the carbon isotope ratios of whole diet and dietary protein to those of bone collagen and carbonate', in Lambert, P and Grupe, G (eds), *Prehistoric Human Bone: Archaeology at the Molecular Level* (Berlin: Springer, 1993)
19. Ambrose and Norr op cit; Lee-Thorp, J A *et al.* 'Stable carbon isotope ratio differences between bone collagen and bone apatite, and their relationship to diet', *J Archaeol Sci* 1989; 16: 585–599
20. Hillman, G 'Late Pleistocene changes in wild plant-foods available to 'hunter-gatherers' of the northern Fertile Crescent: possible preludes to cereal cultivation', in Harris, D R (ed.), *The Origins and Spread of Agriculture and Pastoralism in Eurasia* (London: UCL Press, 1996)
21. Bar-Yosef, O 'Earliest food producers-Prepottery Neolithic (8000–5500)', in Levy, T E (ed.), *The Archaeology of Society in the Holy Land* (Leicester: Leicester University Press, 1995)
22. Cordain, L *et al.* 'Plant-animal subsistence ratios and macronutrient energy estimations in worldwide 'hunter-gatherer' diets', *Am J Clin Nutr* 2000; 71(3): 682–92

Chapter 2

1. Bar-Yosef O and Belfer-Cohen A 'From foraging to farming in the Mediterranean Levant', in Gebauer, A B and Price, T D (eds), *Transitions to Agriculture in Prehistory* (Madison, WI: Prehistory Press, 1992)

2. Molleson, T I *et al.* 'Dietary changes and the effects of food preparation on microwear patterns in the Late Neolithic of Abu Hureyra, northern Syria', *J Hum Evol* 1993; 24: 455–68

3. Goodman, A H *et al.* 'Health changes at Dickson Mounds, Illinois', in Cohen, M N and Armelagos, G J (eds), *Paleopathology and the Origins of Agriculture* (London: Academic Press, 1984)

4. Rose, J C *et al.* 'Paleopathology and the origins of maize agriculture in the Lower Mississippi Valley and Caddoan culture areas', in Cohen, M N and Armelagos, G J (eds), *Paleopathology and the Origins of Agriculture* (London: Academic Press, 1984)

5. Cook, D C 'Subsistence and health in the Lower Illinois Valley: osteological evidence', in Cohen, M N and Armelagos, G J (eds), *Paleopathology and the Origins of Agriculture* (London: Academic Press, 1984)

6. Larsen, C S 'Health and disease in prehistoric Georgia: the transition to agriculture', in Cohen, M N and Armelagos, G J (eds), *Paleopathology and the Origins of Agriculture* (London. Academic Press, 1984)

7. Ubelaker, D H 'Prehistoric human biology of Equador: Possible temporal trends and cultural correlations', in Cohen, M N and Armelagos, G J (eds), *Paleopathology and the Origins of Agriculture* (London: Academic Press, 1984)

8. Norr, L 'Prehistoric subsistence and health status of coastal peoples from the Panamanian Isthmus of Lower Central America', in Cohen, M N and Armelagos, G J (eds), *Paleopathology and the Origins of Agriculture* (London: Academic Press, 1984)

9. Allison, M J 'Paleopathology in Peruvian and Chilean populations', in Cohen, M N and Armelagos, G J (eds), *Paleopathology and the Origins of Agriculture* (London: Academic Press, 1984)

10. Angel, L J 'Health as a crucial factor in the changes from hunting to developed farming in the eastern Mediterranean', in Cohen, M N and Armelagos, G J (eds), *Paleopathology and the Origins of Agriculture* (London: Academic Press, 1984)

11. Cordain, L 'Solved: the 10,000-year-old riddle of bread and milk', *CAM* July 2006; 20–25

12. Angel op cit

Chapter 3

1. Cordain, L *et al.* 'Origins and evolution of the Western diet: health implications for the 21st century', *Am J Clin Nutr* 2005; 81(2): 341–54
2. *National Diet and Nutrition Survey* (The Office of National Statistics, 2004)
3. Galloway, J H 'Sugar', in Kiple, K F and Ornelas, K C (eds), *The Cambridge World History of Food* (vol 1; Cambridge University Press, 2000): 437–49
4. *National Diet and Nutrition Survey* op cit
5. Copley, M S *et al.* Direct chemical evidence for widespread dairying in prehistoric Britain. *Proc Natl Acad Sci USA* 2003; 100: 1524–9
6. *National Diet and Nutrition Survey* op cit
7. McGovern, P E *et al.* 'Neolithic resinated wine', *Nature* 1996; 381: 480–1
8. *National Diet and Nutrition Survey* op cit
9. Kurlansky, M *Salt: a world history* (New York: Walker and Company, 2002)
10. He, F J *et al.* 'Effect of modest salt reduction on blood pressure: a meta-analysis of randomized trials. Implications for public health', *Journal of Human Hypertension* 2002; 16(11): 761–70
11. Simoons, F J 'The geographic hypothesis and lactose malabsorption. A weighing of the evidence', *Am J Dig Dis* 1978; 23(11): 963–80
12. Cordain, L *et al.* 'Plant-animal subsistence ratios and macronutrient energy estimations in worldwide 'hunter-gatherer' diets', *Am J Clin Nutr* 2000; 71(3): 682–92

Chapter 4

1. Cordain, L *et al.* 'Hyperinsulinemic diseases of civilization: more than just Syndrome X', *Comparative Biochemistry and Physiology* 2003 136: 95–112
2. Roberts, S B 'High-glycemic index foods, hunger, and obesity: is there a connection?', *Nutrition Review* 2000 58: 163–9
3. Febbraio, M A *et al.* 'Preexercise carbohydrate ingestion, glucose kinetics, and muscle glycogen use: effect of the glycemic index', *J Appl Physiol* 2000; 89: 1845–51
4. Colditz, G A *et al.* 'Diet and risk of clinical diabetes in women', *Am J Clin Nutr* 1992; 55: 1018–23
5. Collier, G R *et al.* 'Low glycemic index starchy foods improve glucose control and lower serum cholesterol in diabetic children', *Diabetes Nutr Metab* 1988; 1: 11–19

6. Fontvieille, A M *et al.* 'A moderate switch from high to low glycemic-index foods for 3 weeks improves metabolic control of type I (IDDM) diabetic subjects', *Diabetes Nutr Metab* 1988; 1: 139–43

7. Jenkins, D J *et al.* 'Low-glycemic-index starchy foods in the diabetic diet', *Am J Clin Nutr* 1988; 48: 248–54

8. Wolever, T M *et al.* 'Beneficial effect of a low glycaemic index diet in type 2 diabetes', *Diabet Med* 1992; 9: 451–8

9. Wolever, T M *et al.* 'Beneficial effect of low-glycemic index diet in overweight NIDDM subjects', *Diabetes Care* 1992; 15: 562–4

10. Brand, J C *et al.* 'Low-glycemic index foods improve long-term glycemic control in NIDDM', *Diabetes Care* 1991; 14: 95–101

11. Fontvieille, A M *et al.* 'The use of low glycaemic index foods improves metabolic control of diabetic patients over five weeks', *Diabet Med* 1992; 9: 444–50

12. Frost, G *et al.* 'Dietary advice based on the glycaemic index improves dietary profile and metabolic control in type 2 diabetic patients', *Diabet Med* 1994; 11: 397–401

13. GI Table adapted from Foster-Powell K *et al.* 'International table of glycemic index and glycemic load values', *Am J Clin Nutr* 2002; 76(1): 5–56

14. Feinman, R D *et al.* 'Thermodynamics and metabolic advantage of weight loss diets', *Metabolic Syndrome and Related Disorders* 2003; 1: 209–109

15. Bier, D M 'The energy cost of protein metabolism: lean and mean on Uncle Sam's team', in *The role of protein and amino acids in sustaining and enhancing performance* (Washington, DC: National Academies Press, 1999): 109–19

16. Hue, L 'Regulation of gluconeogenesis in liver', In Jefferson, L and Cherrington, A (eds), *Handbook of physiology: the endocrine system* (Oxford: Oxford University Press, 2001)

17. Foster-Powell *et al.*, op cit.

18. Slabber, M *et al.* 'Effects of a low-insulin-response, energy-restricted diet on weight loss and plasma insulin concentrations in hyperinsulinemic obese females', *Am J Clin Nutr* 1994; 60: 48–53

19. Spieth, L E *et al.* 'A low-glycemic index diet in the treatment of pediatric obesity', *Arch Pediatr Adolesc Med* 2000; 154: 947–51

20. Clapp, J R 'Diet, exercise and feto-placental growth', *Arch Gynecol Obstet* 1997; 261: 101–7

21. Bravata, D M *et al.* 'Efficacy and safety of low-carbohydrate diets a systematic review', *JAMA* 2003; 289(14): 1837–1850

22. Brehm, B J *et al.* 'A randomized trial comparing a very low carbohydrate diet and a calorie-restricted low fat diet on body weight and cardiovascular risk factors in healthy women', *J Clin Endocrinol Metab* 2003; 88: 1617–23

23. Foster, G D *et al.* 'A randomized trial of a low-carbohydrate diet for obesity', *N Engl J Med* 2003; 348: 2082–90

24. Yancy, W S Jr *et al.* 'A low carbohydrate, ketogenic diet versus a low-fat diet to treat obesity and hyperlipidemia. A randomized, controlled trial', *Ann Intern Med* 2004; 140: 69–77

25. Stern, L *et al.* 'The effects of low-carbohydrate versus conventional weight loss diets in severely obese adults: one-year follow-up of a randomized trial', *Ann Intern Med* 2004; 140: 778–85

26. Foster, op cit

27. Stern., op cit

28. Ibid.

29. Foster, op cit

30. Bravata, op cit

31. Johnston, C S *et al.* 'Ketogenic low-carbohydrate diets have no metabolic advantage over nonketogenic low-carbohydrate diets', *Am J Clin Nutr* 2006 83: 1055–61

32. Yancy, op cit

33. Brehm, op cit

34. Farnsworth, E *et al.* 'Effect of a high-protein, energy-restricted diet on body composition, glycemic control, and lipid concentrations in overweight and obese hyperinsulinemic men and women', *Am J Clin Nutr* 2003; 78: 31–9.

35. Foster, op cit

36. Meckling, K A *et al.* 'Comparison of a low-fat diet to a low-carbohydrate diet on weight loss, body composition, and risk factors for diabetes and cardio-vascular disease in free-living, overweight men and women', *J Clin Endocrinol Metab* 2004; 89: 2717–23

37. Sharman, M J *et al.* 'A ketogenic diet favorably affects serum biomarkers for cardiovascular disease in normal-weight men', *J Nutr* 2002; 132: 1879–85

38. Sharman, M J *et al.* 'Very low-carbohydrate and low-fat diets affect fasting lipids and postprandial lipemia differently in overweight men', *J Nutr* 2004; 134: 880–5

39. Volek, J S *et al.* 'An isoenergetic very low carbohydrate diet improves serum HDL cholesterol and triacylglycerol concentrations, the total cholesterol to HDL cholesterol ratio and postpranthal lipemic responses compared with a

low fat diet in normal weight, normolipidemic women', *JNutr* 2003; 133: 2756–61

40. Volek, J S *et al.* 'Comparison of a very low-carbohydrate and low-fat diet on fasting lipids, LDL subclasses, insulin resistance, and postprandial lipemic responses in overweight women', *JAm Coil Nutr* 2004; 23: 177–84

41. Halton, T L *et al.* 'Low-carbohydrate-diet score and risk of coronary heart disease in women', *N Engl J Med* 2006; 355: 1991–2002

42. Manninen, A H 'High-protein weight loss diets and purported adverse effects: where is the evidence?', *Sports Nutrition Review Journal* 2004; 1(1): 45–51

43. Drewnowski, A 'Concept of a nutritious food: toward a nutrient density score', *Am J Clin Nutr* 2005 82: 721–32

44. Fuchs, C S *et al.* 'Dietary fiber and the risk of colorectal cancer and adenoma in women', *N Engl J Med* 1999; 340(3): 169–76

45. Jacobs, E T *et al.* 'Intake of supplemental and total fiber and risk of colorectal adenoma recurrence in the wheat bran fiber trial', *Cancer Epidemiol Biomarkers Prev* 2002 11(9): 906–14

46. Alberts, D S *et al.* 'Lack of effect of a high-fiber cereal supplement on the recurrence of colorectal adenomas. Phoenix Colon Cancer Prevention Physicians' Network', *N Engl J Med* 2000; 342(16): 1156–62

47. Shattock, P *et al.* 'Biochemical aspects in autism spectrum disorders: updating the opioid-excess theory and presenting new opportunities for biomedical intervention', *Expert Opin Ther Targets* 2002 6(2): 175–83

48. Millward, C *et al.* 'Gluten- and casein-free diets for autistic spectrum disorder', *Cochrane Database Syst Rev* 2004; (2): CD003498, Knivsber, A M *et al.* 'Reports on dietary intervention in autistic disorders', *Nutr Neurosci* 2001; 4(1): 25–37

49. Janatuinen, E K *et al.* 'No harm from five year ingestion of oats in coeliac disease', *Gut* 2002 50(3): 332–5

50. Hogberg, L *et al.* 'Oats to children with newly diagnosed coeliac disease: a randomised double blind study', *Gut* 2004 53(5): 649–54

Chapter 5

1. Brynes, A E *et al.* 'A randomised four-intervention crossover study investigating the effect of carbohydrates on daytime profiles of insulin, glucose, non-esterified fatty acids and triacylglycerols in middle-aged men', *British Journal of Nutrition* 2003; 89: 207–18

2. Ludwig, D S *et al.* 'Relation between consumption of sugar-sweetened drinks and childhood obesity: a prospective, observational analysis', *Lancet* 2001 357: 505–8

3. Sanchez, A *et al.* 'Role of Sugars in Human Neutrophilic Phagocytosis', *Am J Clin Nutr* Nov 1973; 261: 1180–4

4. Bernstein, J *et al.* 'Depression of Lymphocyte Transformation Following Oral Glucose Ingestion', *Am J Clin Nutr* 1997; 30: 613

5. Ringsdorf, W *et al.* 'Sucrose, Neutrophilic Phagocytosis and Resistance to Disease', *Dental Survey* 1976; 52(12): 46–8

6. Couzy, F *et al.* 'Nutritional Implications of the Interaction Minerals', *Progressive Food and Nutrition Science* 17; 1933: 65–87

7. Kozlovsky, A *et al.* 'Effects of Diets High in Simple Sugars on Urinary Chromium Losses', *Metabolism* 1986; 35: 515–18

8. Fields, M *et al.* 'Effect of Copper Deficiency on Metabolism and Mortality in Rats Fed Sucrose or Starch Diets', *Journal of Clinical Nutrition* 1983; 113: 1335–45

9. Lemann, J 'Evidence that Glucose Ingestion Inhibits Net Renal Tubular Reabsorption of Calcium and Magnesium', *Journal of Clinical Nutrition* 1976; 70: 236–45

10. Reiser, S *et al.* 'Effects of Sugars on Indices on Glucose Tolerance in Humans', *Am J Clin Nutr* 1986; 43: 151–59

11. Schulze, MB *et al.* 'Sugar-sweetened beverages, weight gain, and incidence of type 2 diabetes in young and middle-aged women. *JAMA* 2004; 292(8): 927–34

12. Official Dietary Reference Intakes for energy, carbohydrate, fibre, fat, fatty acids, cholesterol, protein and amino acids (US Institute of Medicine, 2002)

13. *Report of a Joint FAO/WHO Consultation: Carbohydrates in human nutrition*, FAO Food and Nutrition Paper 66 (Geneva: World Health Organization, 1998)

14. news.bbc.co.uk/1/hi/health/3726510.stm

15. news.bbc.co.uk/nol/shared/spl/hi/programmes/panorama/transcripts/the troublewithsugar.txt

16. Elliott, S S *et al.* 'Fructose, weight gain and the insulin resistance syndrome', *Am J Clin Nutr* 2002 76(5): 911–22

17. Kavet, R *et al.* 'The Toxicity of Inhaled Methanol Vapors', *Critical Reviews in Toxicology* 1990 21; 1: 21–50

18. Trocho, C *et al.* 'Formaldehyde Derived from Dietary Aspartame Binds to Tissue Components in vivo', *Life Sciences* 1998 63; 5: 337

19. Main, D M *et al.* 'Health Effects of Low-Level Exposure to Formaldehyde', *Journal of Occupational Medicine* 1983; 25: 896–900
20. Olsen, J H *et al.* 'Formaldehyde induced symptoms in day care centers', *American Industrial Hygiene Association Journal* 43; 5 366–70
21. Burdach, S *et al.* 'Damages to health in schools. Complaints caused by the use of formaldehyde-emitting materials in school buildings', *Fortschritte Med* 1980 98 11; 379–84
22. Main, op cit
23. Burdach, op cit
24. Kilburn, K H *et al.* 'Neurobehavioral and respiratory symptoms of formaldehyde and xylene exposure in histology technicians', *Arch Env Health* 1985 40; 4; 229–33
25. Camfield, P R *et al.* 'Aspartame exacerbates EEG spike-wave discharge in children with generalized absence epilepsy: a double-blind controlled study', *Neurology* 1992; 42: 1000–3
26. Walton, R G *et al.* 'Adverse reactions to aspartame: double-blind challenge in patients from a vulnerable population', *Biol Psychiatry* 1993; 34(1–2): 13–17
27. Van Den Eeden, S K *et al.* 'Aspartame Ingestion and Headaches: A Randomized, Crossover Trial', *Neurology* 1994; 44: 1787–93
28. Lipton, R B *et al.* 'Aspartame as a dietary trigger of headache', *Headache* 1989; 29(2): 90–2
29. www.dorway.com/peerrev.html
30. Soffritti, M *et al.* 'First experimental demonstration of the multipotential carcinogenic effects of aspartame administered in the feed to Sprague-Dawley rats', *Environ Health Perspect* 2006; Mar; 114(3): 379–85
31. Lavin, J H *et al.* 'The Effect of Sucrose- and Aspartame-Sweetened Drinks on Energy Intake, Hunger and Food Choice of Female, Moderately Restrained Eaters', *Int J Obes* 1997; 21: 37–42
32. Tordoff, M G *et al.* 'Oral stimulation with aspartame increases hunger', *Physiol Behav* 1990; 47: 555–9

Chapter 6

1. Lanou, A J *et al.* 'Calcium, dairy products, and bone health in children and young adults: a reevaluation of the evidence', *Pediatrics* 2005; 115(3): 736–43
2. Winzenberg, T *et al.* 'Effects of calcium supplementation on bone density in healthy children: meta-analysis of randomised controlled trials', *BMJ* 2006; 333: 775–8

3. Lanou, A J 'Bone health in children', *BMJ* 2006; 333: 763–4

4. Feskanich, D *et al.* 'Calcium, vitamin D, milk consumption, and hip fractures: a prospective study among postmenopausal women', *Am J Clin Nutr* 2003 77(2): 504–11

5. Weinsier, R L *et al.* 'Dairy foods and bone health: examination of the evidence', *Am J Clin Nutr* 2000; 72: 681–9

6. Loones, A 'Transformation of milk components during yogurt fermentation', in Chandan, R C (ed.), *Yoghurt: nutritional and health properties* (McClean, VA: National Yoghurt Association, 1989): 95–114

7. Beshkova, D M *et al.* 'Production of amino acids by yoghurt bacteria', *Biotechnol Prog* 1998; 14: 963–5

8. Wang, G J *et al.* 'Gastric stimulation in obese subjects activates the hippocampus and other regions involved in brain reward circuitry', *PNAS* 2006; 103: 15641–5

Chapter 7

1. Cordain, L *et al.* 'Fatty acid analysis of wild ruminant tissues: evolutionary implications for reducing diet-related chronic disease', *Eur J Clin Nutr* 2002; 56: 181–91; Eaton, S B and Konner, M 'Paleolithic nutrition. A consideration of its nature and current implications', *N Engl J Med* 1985; 312: 283–9

2. Simopoulos, A P and Cleland, L G (eds) 'Omega-6/omega-3 Essential Fatty Acid Ratio: The Scientific Evidence', *World Rev Nutr Diet*. Basel, Karger, 2003, Vol 92

3. Weber, P C 'Are we what we eat? Fatty acids in nutrition and in cell membranes: cell functions and disorders induced by dietary conditions', in *Fish fats and your health* (Norway: Svanoy Foundation, 1989): 9–18

4. Raheja, B S *et al.* 'Significance of the n-6/n-3 ratio for insulin action in diabetes', *Ann NY Acad Sci* 1993; 683: 258–71

5. Simopoulos, A P 'The importance of the ratio of omega-6/omega-3 essential fatty acids', *Biomed Pharmacother* 2002; 56(8): 365–79

6. Pedersen, J I *et al.* 'Adipose tissue fatty acids and risk of myocardial infarction – A case-control study', *Eur J Clin Nutr* 2000; 54: 618–25

7. Ascherio, A *et al.* 'Dietary fat and risk of coronary heart disease in men: Cohort follow up study in the United States', *BMJ* 1996; 313: 84–90

8. Hu, F B *et al.* 'Dietary fat intake and the risk of coronary heart disease in women', *N Engl J Med* 1997; 337: 1491–9

9. Oomen, C M *et al.* 'Association between trans fatty acid intake and 10–year

risk of coronary heart disease in the Zutphen Elderly Study: A prospective population-based study', *Lancet* 2001; 357: 746–51

10. Bakker, N *et al.* 'The Euramic Study Group: Adipose fatty acids and cancers of the breast, prostate and colon: An ecological study', *Cancer* 1997; 72: 587–97

11. Christiansen, E *et al.* 'Intake of a diet high in trans monounsaturated fatty acids or saturated fatty acids. Effects on postprandial insulinemia and glycemia in obese patients with NIDDM', *Diabetes Care* 1997; 20: 881–7

12. Alstrup, K K *et al.* 'Differential effects of cis and *trans* fatty acids on insulin release from isolated mouse islets', *Metabolism* 1999; 48: 22–9

13. Salméron, J *et al.* 'Dietary fat intake and risk of type 2 diabetes in women', *Am J Clin Nutr* 2001; 73: 1019–26

14. Kavanagh, K *et al.* 'Trans fat diet induces insulin resistance in monkeys', Study presented at the Scientific Sessions of the American Diabetes Association in Washington DC, 2006

15. Williams, M A *et al.* 'Risk of preeclampsia in relation to elaidic acid (trans fatty acid) in maternal erythrocytes', *Gynecol Obstet Invest* 1998; 46: 84–7

16. Elias, S L *et al.* 'Infant plasma trans. n-6, and n-3 fatty acids and conjugated linoleic acids are related to maternal plasma fatty acids, length of gestation, and birth weight and length', *Am J Clin Nutr* 2001; 73: 807–14

17. Hulshof, K F. 'Intake of fatty acids in western Europe with emphasis on trans fatty acids: the TRANSFAIR Study', *Eur J Clin Nutr* 1999; 53(2): 143–57

18. Letter Report on Dietary Reference Intakes for Trans Fatty Acids, Food and Nutrition Board, Institute of Medicine 10th July 2002

19. Pietinen, P *et al.* 'Intake of fatty acids and risk of coronary heart disease in a cohort of Finnish men. The alpha-tocopherol, beta-carotene cancer prevention trial', *Am J Epidemiol* 1997; 145: 876–87

20. Willett, W C *et al.* 'Intake of fatty acids and risk of coronary heart diseases among women', *Lancet* 1993; 341: 581–5

Chapter 8

1. Lean, M E *et al.* 'Weight loss with high and low carbohydrate 1200 kcal diets in free living women', *Eur J Clin Nutr* 1997; 51: 243–8

2. Wien, M A *et al.* 'Almonds vs complex carbohydrates in a weight reduction program', *Int J Obes* 2003; 27: 1365–72

3. Young, C M *et al.* 'Effect of body composition and other parameters in obese young men of carbohydrate level of reduction diet', *Am J Clin Nutr* 1971; 24: 290–6

4. Fraser, G E *et al.* 'Effect on body weight of a free 76 Kilojoule (320 calorie) daily supplement of almonds for six months', *J Am Coll Nutr* 2002; 21(3): 275–83

5. Sheppard, L *et al.* 'Weight loss in women participating in a randomized trial of low-fat diets', *Am J Clin Nutr* 1991; 54: 821–8

6. Kasim, S E *et al.* 'Dietary and anthropometric determinants of plasma lipoproteins during a long-term low-fat diet in healthy women', *Am J Clin Nutr* 1993; 57: 146–53

7. Jeffery, R W *et al.* 'A randomized trial of counselling for fat restriction versus calorie restriction in the treatment of obesity', Int J Obes 1995; 19: 132–7

8. Pirozzo, S *et al.* 'Advice on low-fat diets for obesity', Cochrane Database Syst Rev. 2002; (2): CD003640

9. Willett, C *et al.* 'Dietary fat is not a major determinant of body fat', *Am J Med* 2002; 113(9B): 47S–59S

10. Keys, A 'Atherosclerosis: a problem in new public health', *Journal of Mount Sinai Hospital* 1953; 20: 118–39

11. Keys, A. 'Coronary heart disease in seven countries', *Circulation* 1970; 41 (supplement 1): 1–211

12. Paul, O *et al.* 'A longitudinal study of coronary heart disease', *Circulation*, Jul 1963; 28: 20–31

13. Gordon, T. 'The Framingham Diet Study: diet and the regulation of serum cholesterol', in *The Framingham Study: An Epidemiological Investigation of Cardiovascular Disease*, Section 24 (US Government Printing Office, Washington, DC, 1970)

14. Medalie, J H *et al.* 'Five-year myocardial infarction incidence. II. Association of single variables to age and birthplace', *Journal of Chronic Diseases* June 1973; 26 (6): 325–49

15. Morris, I N *et al.* 'Diet and heart: a postscript', *BMJ* 1977; 2: 1307–14

16. Yano, K *et al.* 'Dietary intake and the risk of coronary heart disease in Japanese men living in Hawaii', *Am J Clin Nutr* Jul 1978; 31: 1270–9

17. Garcia-Palmieri, M R *et al.* 'Relationship of dietary intake to subsequent coronary heart disease incidence: The Puerto Rico Heart Health Program', *Am J Clin Nutr* Aug 1980; 33 (8): 1818–27

18. Gordon, T *et al.* 'Diet and its relation to coronary heart disease in three populations', *Circulation* Mar 1981; 63; 500–15

19. Shekelle, R B *et al.* 'Diet, serum cholesterol, and death from coronary heart disease: the Western Electric Study', *N Engl J Med* 1981; 304: 65–70

20. McGee, D L *et al.* 'Ten-year incidence of coronary heart disease in the Honolulu Heart Program: relationship to nutrient intake', *American Journal of Epidemiology* 1984; 119: 667–76

21. Kromhout, D *et al.* 'Diet, prevalence and 10–year mortality from coronary heart disease in 871 middle-aged men: the Zutphen Study', *American Journal of Epidemiology* 1984; 119: 733–41

22. Kushi, L H *et al.* 'Diet and 20–year mortality from coronary heart disease: the Ireland-Boston Diet-Heart Study', *N Engl J Med* 1985; 312: 811–18

23. Lapidus, L *et al.* 'Dietary habits in relation to incidence of cardiovascular disease and death in women: a 12–year follow-up of participants in the population study of women in Gothenburg, Sweden', *Am J Clin Nutr* Oct 1986; 44(4): 444–8

24. Khaw, K T *et al.* 'Dietary fiber and reduced ischemic heart disease mortality rates in men and women: a 12–year prospective study', *American Journal of Epidemiology* Dec 1987; 126 (6): 1093–1102

25. Farchi, G *et al.* 'Diet and 20–y mortality in two rural population groups of middle-aged men in Italy', *Am J Clin Nutr* Nov 1989; 50 (5): 1095–1103

26. Posner, B M *et al.* 'Dietary lipid predictors of coronary heart disease in men: the Framingham Study', *Arch Int Med* 1991; 151: 1181–7

27. Dolecek, T A. 'Epidemiological evidence of relationships between dietary polyunsaturated fatty acids and mortality in the multiple risk factor intervention trial', *Proceedings of the Society for Experimental Biology and Medicine,* Jun 1992; 200 (2): 177–82

28. Fehily, A M *et al.* 'Diet and incident ischaemic heart disease: the Caerphilly Study', *British Journal of Nutrition* 1993; 69: 303–14

29. Goldbourt, U *et al.* 'Factors predictive of long-term coronary heart disease mortality among 10,059 male Israeli civil servants and municipal employees: a 23-year mortality follow-up in the Israeli Ischemic Heart Disease Study', *Cardiology* 1993; 82: 100–21

30. Esrey, K L *et al.* 'Relationship between dietary intake and coronary heart disease mortality: Lipid Research Clinics Prevalence Follow-Up Study', *Journal of Clinical Epidemiology* Feb 1996; 49 (2): 211–16

31. Ascherio, A *et al.* 'Dietary fat and risk of coronary heart disease in men: cohort follow-up study in the United States', *BMJ* 1996; 313: 84–90

32. Pietinen, P *et al.* 'Intake of fatty acids and risk of coronary heart disease in a cohort of Finnish men: the Aipha-Tocopherol, Beta-Carotene Cancer Prevention Study', *American Journal of Epidemiology* 1997; 145: 876–87

33. Hu, F B *et al.* 'Dietary fat intake and the risk of coronary heart disease in women', *N Engl J Med* Nov 20, 1997; 337 (21): 1491–9

34. Tanasescu, M *et al.* 'Dietary fat and cholesterol and the risk of cardiovascular disease among women with type 2 diabetes', *Am J Clin Nutr* Jun 2004; 79: 999–1005

35. Laaksonen, D E *et al.* 'Prediction of cardiovascular mortality in middle-aged men by dietary and serum linoleic and polyunsaturated fatty acids', *Arch Int Med* 2005; 165: 193–9

36. Tucker, K L *et al.* 'The Combination of High Fruit and Vegetable and Low Saturated Fat Intakes Is More Protective against Mortality in Aging Men than Is Either Alone: The Baltimore Longitudinal Study of Aging', *Journal of Nutrition* 2005; 135: 556–61

37. Leosdottir, M *et al.* 'Dietary fat intake and early mortality patterns – data from The Malmo Diet and Cancer Study', *Journal of Internal Medicine* 2005; 258: 153–65.

38. The four studies were McGee, op cit; Kushi, op cit; Esrey, op cit and Tucker, op cit.

39. Mozaffarian, D *et al.* 'Dietary fats, carbohydrate, and progression of coronary atherosclerosis in postmenopausal women', *Am J Clin Nutr* 2004; 80(5): 1175–84

40. Yusuf, S *et al.* 'Effect of potentially modifiable risk factors associated with myocardial infarction in 52 countries (the INTERHEART study): case-control study', *Lancet* 2004; 364(9438): 937–52

41. Dayton, S *et al.* 'A controlled clinical trial of a diet high in unsaturated fat in preventing complications of atherosclerosis', *Circulation* 1969; 40 (Suppl. II): 1–63

42. Frantz, I D Jr *et al.* 'Test of effect of lipid lowering by diet on cardiovascular risk. The Minnesota coronary survey', *Arteriosclerosis* 1989; 9: 129–35

43. Key TJ, et al. Mortality in British vegetarians review and preliminary results from EPIC-Oxford. Am J Clin Nutr 2003; 78(suppl): 533S-8S

44. Key TJA, et al. Dietary habits and mortality in 11,000 vegetarians and health-conscious people: results of a 17-year follow up. BMJ 1996; 313: 775–9

45. Thorogood M, et al. Risk of death from cancer and ischemic heart disease in meat and non-meat eaters. BMJ 1994; 308: 1667–70

46. Rose, G A *et al.* 'Corn oil in treatment of ischaemic heart disease', *BMJ* 1965; 1: 1531–3

47. Christakis, G *et al.* 'Effect of the Anti-Coronary Club on coronary heart disease risk factor status', *JAMA* 1966; 198 (6): 597–604

48. Bierenbaum, M L *et al.* 'Modified fat dietary management of the young male with coronary disease. A five year-report', *JAMA* 1967; 202(13): 1119–23

49. 'National Diet Heart Study. Final report', *Circulation* 1968; 37(3 Suppl): 1–428

50. 'Controlled trial of soya-bean oil in myocardial infarction', *Lancet* 1968; 2(9757): 693–9

51. Leren, P 'The Oslo Diet-Heart Study: Eleven Year Report', *Circulation* 1970; 42: 935–42

52 Miettinen, M *et al.* 'Effect of cholesterol-lowering diet on mortality from coronary heart disease and other causes. A twelve-year clinical trial in men and women', *Lancet* 1972; 2(7782): 835–8

53. Woodhill, J M *et al.* 'Low fat, low cholesterol diet in secondary prevention of coronary heart disease', *Advances in Experimental Medicine and Biology* 1978; 109: 317–30

54. Turpenien, O *et al.* 'Dietary prevention of coronary heart disease: the Finnish Mental Hospital Study', *Int J Epidemiol* 1979; 8: 9–118

55. Hjermann, I *et al.* 'Effect of diet and smoking in the incidence of coronary heart disease', *Lancet* 1981; ii: 1303–10

56. World Health Organization European Collaborative Group, 'European collaborative trial of multifactorial prevention of coronary heart disease', *Lancet* 1986; 1: 869–72

57. Burr, M L *et al.* 'Effects of changes in fat, fish, and fibre intakes on death and myocardial reinfarction: diet and reinfarction trial (DART)', *Lancet* 1989; 2(8666): 757–61

58. Strandberg, T E *et al.* 'Long-term mortality after 5 year multifactorial primary prevention of cardiovascular diseases in middle-aged men', *JAMA* 1991; 266: 1229

59. Watts, G F *et al.* 'Effects on coronary artery disease of lipid-lowering diet, or diet plus cholestyramine, in the St Thomas' atherosclerosis regression study (STARS)', *Lancet* 1992; 339(8793): 563–9

60. Neaton, J D *et al.* 'Serum cholesterol level and mortality: findings for men screened in the Multiple Risk Factor Intervention Trial', *Arch Int Med* 1992; 152: 1490–1500

61. De Lorgeril, M *et al.* 'Mediterranean alpha-linolenic acid-rich diet in secondary prevention of coronary heart disease', *Lancet*, 1994; 343(8911): 1454–9

62. Howard, B V *et al.* 'Low-Fat Dietary Pattern and Risk of Cardiovascular Disease: The Women's Health Initiative Randomized Controlled Dietary Modification Trial', *JAMA* 2006; 295: 655–66

63. Morrison, op cit; Hood, op cit; Miettinen, op cit; Turpenien, op cit; Watts, op cit; De Lorgeril, op cit

64. Morrison, op cit

65. Watts, op cit; De Lorgeril, op cit

66. Hooper, L *et al.* 'Dietary intake and prevention of cardiovascular disease: systematic review', *BMJ* 2001; 322(7289): 757–63

67. Lawson, L D *et al.* 'Beta-oxidation of the coenzyme A esters of elaidic, oleic and stearic acids and their full-cycle intermediates by rat heart mitochondria', *Biochem Biophys Acta* 1979; 573: 245–54

68. Hassig, C A *et al.* 'Fiber-derived butyrate and the prevention of colon cancer', *Chem Biol* 1997; 4: 783–9

69. Burton, A F 'Oncolytic effects of fatty acids in mice and rats', *Am J Clin Nutr* 1991; 53(suppl): 1082–6

70. Thormar, H *et al.* 'Inactivation of visna virus and other enveloped viruses by free fatty acids and monoglycerides', *Ann NY Acad Sci* l994; 724: 465–71

71. Neyts, J *et al.* 'Hydrogels containing monocaprin prevent intravaginal and intracutaneous infections with HSV-2 in mice: impact on the search for vaginal microbicides', *J Med Virol* 2000; 61: 107–10

72. Dawson, P L *et al.* 'Effect of lauric acid and nisin-impregnated soy-based films on the growth of *Listeria monocytogenes* on turkey bologna', *Poult Sci* 2002; 81: 721–6

73. Sun, C Q *et al.* 'The antimicrobial properties of milkfat after partial hydrolysis by calf pregastric lipase', *Chem Biol interact* 2002; 140: 185–98

74. Scientific steering committee on behalf of the Simon Broome Register group. 'Risk of fatal coronary heart disease in familial hypercholesterolaemia', *BMJ* 1991; 303: 893–6

75. Forette, F *et al.* 'The prognostic significance of isolated systolic hypertension in the elderly. Results of a ten year longitudinal survey', *Clinical and Experimental Hypertension* Part A, Theory and Practice, 1982; 4: 1177–91

76. Siegel, D *et al.* 'Predictors of cardiovascular events and mortality in the Systolic Hypertension in the Elderly Program pilot project', *American Journal of Epidemiology* 1987; 126: 385–9

77. Nissinen, A *et al.* 'Risk factors for cardiovascular disease among 55 to 74 year-old Finnish men: a 10-year follow-up', *Annals of Medicine* 1989; 21: 239–40

78. Krumholz, H M *et al.* 'Lack of association between cholesterol and coronary heart disease mortality and morbidity and all-cause mortality in persons older than 70 years', *JAMA* 1994; 272: 1335–40

79. Weijenberg, M P *et al.* 'Serum total cholesterol and systolic blood pressure as risk factors for mortality from ischemic heart disease among elderly men and women', *Journal of Clinical Epidemiology* 1994; 47: 197–205

80. Simons, L A *et al.* 'Diabetes, mortality and coronary heart disease in the prospective Dubbo study of Australian elderly', *Australian and New Zealand Journal of Medicine* 1996; 26: 66–74

81. Weijenberg, M P *et al.* 'Total and high density lipoprotein cholesterol as risk factors for coronary heart disease in elderly men during 5 years of follow-up. The Zutphen Elderly Study', *American Journal of Epidemiology* 1996; 143: 151–8

82. Simons, L A *et al.* 'Cholesterol and other lipids predict coronary heart disease and ischaemic stroke in the elderly, but only in those below 70 years', *Atherosclerosis* 2001; 159: 201–8

83. Abbott, R D *et al.* 'Age-related changes in risk factor effects on the incidence of coronary heart disease', *Annals of Epidemiology* 2002; 12: 173–81

84. Zimetbaum, P *et al.* 'Plasma lipids and lipoproteins and the incidence of cardiovascular disease in the very elderly. The Bronx aging study', *Arteriosclerosis Thrombosis and Vascular Biology* 1992; 12: 416–23

85. Fried, L P *et al.* 'Risk factors for 5-year mortality in older adults: the Cardiovascular Health Study', *JAMA* 1998; 279: 585–92

86. Chyou, P H *et al.* 'Serum cholesterol concentrations and all-cause mortality in older people', *Age and Ageing* 2000; 29: 69–74

87. Menotti, A *et al.* 'Cardiovascular risk factors and 10-year all-cause mortality in elderly European male populations; the FINE study', *European Heart Journal* 2001; 22: 573–9

88. Räihä, I *et al.* 'Effect of serum lipids, lipoproteins, and apolipoproteins on vascular and nonvascular mortality in the elderly', *Arteriosclerosis Thrombosis and Vascular Biology* 1997; 17: 1224–32

89. Brescianini, S *et al.* 'Low total cholesterol and increased risk of dying: are low levels clinical warning signs in the elderly? Results from the Italian Longitudinal Study on Aging', *Journal of the American Geriatrics Society* 2003; 51(7): 991–6

90. Forette, B *et al.* 'Cholesterol as risk factor for mortality in elderly women', *Lancet* 1989; 1: 868–70

91. Jonsson, A *et al.* 'Total cholesterol and mortality after age 80 years', *Lancet* 1997; 350: 1778–9

92. Weverling-Rijnsburger, A W *et al.* 'Total cholesterol and risk of mortality in the oldest old', *Lancet* 1997; 350: 1119–23

93. Studer, M *et al.* 'Effect of different antilipidemic agents and diets on mortality', *Arch Int Med* 2005; 165: 725–30

94. Thavendiranathan, P *et al.* 'Primary prevention of cardiovascular diseases with statin therapy: a meta-analysis of randomized controlled trials', *Arch Int Med* 2006; 166(21): 2307–13

95. Manuel, D G *et al.* 'Effectiveness and efficiency of different guidelines on statin treatment for preventing deaths from coronary heart disease: modeling study', *BMJ* 2006; 332: 1419 (17 June), doi: 10.1136/*BMJ*.38849.487546.DE

96. Hayward, R A *et al.* 'Narrative review: lack of evidence for recommended low-density lipoprotein treatment targets: a solvable problem', *Ann Int Med* 2006; 145: 520–30

97. Gillman, M W *et al.* 'Margarine intake and subsequent coronary heart disease in men', *Epidemiology* 1997; 8(2): 144–9

Chapter 9

1. *McCance and Widdowson's The Composition of Foods* (Food Standards Agency UK)

2. Astrup, A. 'The satiating power of protein – a key to obesity prevention', *Am J Clin Nutr* 2005; 82(1): 1–2

3. Bier, D M. 'The energy cost of protein metabolism: lean and mean on Uncle Sam's team', in *The role of protein and amino acids in sustaining and enhancing performance* (Washington, DC: National Academies Press, 1999): 109–19

4. Weigle, D S *et al.* 'A high-protein diet induces sustained reductions in appetite, ad libitum caloric intake, and body weight despite compensatory changes in diurnal plasma leptin and ghrelin concentrations', *Am J Clin Nutr* 2005; 82: 41–8

5. Krieger, J W *et al.* 'Effects of variation in protein and carbohydrate intake on body mass and composition during energy restriction', *Am J Clin Nutr* 2006; 83(2): 260–74

6. Devine, A *et al.* 'Protein consumption is an important predictor of lower limb bone mass in elderly women', *Am J Clin Nutr* 2005; 81: 1423–8

7. Ponnampalam, E N *et al.* 'Effect of feeding systems on omega-3 fatty acids, conjugated linoleic acid and trans fatty acids in Australian beef cuts: potential impact on human health', *Asia Pac J Clin Nutr* 2006; 15(1): 21–9

8. Engel, L S *et al.* 'Population Attributable Risks of Esophageal and Gastric Cancers', *Journal of the National Cancer Institute* 2003; 95(18): 1404–13

9. Sarasua, S *et al.* 'Cured and broiled meat consumption in relation to childhood cancer: Denver, Colorado (United States)', *Cancer Causes Control* 1994 Mar; 5(2): 141–8

10. Truswell, A S. 'Meat consumption and cancer of the large bowel', *Eur J Clin Nutr* 2002 Mar; (Suppl 1): 19–24

11. Norat, T *et al.* 'Meat consumption and colorectal cancer risk: dose-response meta-analysis of epidemiological studies', *Int J Cancer* 2002; 98(2): 241–56

12. Larsson, S C *et al.* 'Meat consumption and risk of colorectal cancer: a meta-analysis of prospective studies', *Int J Cancer* 2006; 119(11): 2657–64

13. Kritchevsky, S B *et al.* 'Egg consumption and coronary heart disease: an epidemiological overview', *Journal of the American College of Nutrition* 2000; 19(5): 549–55

14. Wang, C *et al.* 'n–3 Fatty acids from fish or fish-oil supplements, but not -linolenic acid, benefit cardiovascular disease outcomes in primary- and secondary-prevention studies: a systematic review', *Am J Clin Nutr* 2006; 84: 5–17

15. Schaefer, E J *et al.* 'Plasma Phosphatidylcholine Docosahexaenoic Acid Content and Risk of Dementia and Alzheimer Disease: The Framingham Heart Study', *Archives of Neurology* 2006; 63: 1545–50

16. Mozaffarian, D *et al.* 'Fish Intake, Contaminants, and Human Health: Evaluating the Risks and the Benefits', *JAMA* 2006; 296: 1885–99

17. World Cancer Research Fund, American Institute for Cancer Research. 'Food, nutrition, and the prevention of cancer: a global perspective', (Washington, DC: American Institute for Cancer Research, 1997)

18. Holt, S H *et al.* 'A satiety index of common foods', *Eur J Clin Nutr* 1995; 49(9): 675–90

19. Key, T J A *et al.* 'Dietary habits and mortality in 11,000 vegetarians and health conscious people: results of a 17-year follow-up', *BMJ* 1996; 313: 775–9

20. La Vecchia, C *et al.* 'Vegetable consumption and risk of chronic disease', *Epidemiology* 1998; 9: 208–10

21. New, S A. 'The role of the skeleton in acid-base homeostasis', *Proceedings of the Nutrition Society* 2002; 61: 151–64

22. Hu, F B *et al.* 'Frequent nut consumption and risk of coronary heart disease in women: prospective cohort study', *BMJ* 1998 Nov 14; 317(7169): 1341–5

23. Albert, C M *et al.* 'Nut consumption and decreased risk of sudden cardiac

death in the Physicians' Health Study', *Arch Intern Med* 2002 Jun 24; 162(12): 1382–7

24. Alper, C M *et al.* 'Effects of chronic peanut consumption on energy balance and hedonics', *Int J Obes Relat Metab Disord* 2002; 26(8): 1129–37

25. Garcia-Lorda, P *et al.* 'Nut consumption, body weight and insulin resistance', *Eur J Clin Nutr* 57, S8–S11

26. Lajolo, F M *et al.* 'Nutritional significance of lectins and enzyme inhibitors from legumes', *J Agric Food Chem* 2002; 50(22): 6592–8

27. World Cancer Research Fund/American Institute for Cancer Research 'Food, nutrition and the prevention of cancer: a global perspective', (Washington, DC: American Institute for Cancer Research, 1997)

28. Darmadi-Blackberry, I *et al.* 'Legumes: the most important dietary predictor of survival in older people of different ethnicities', *Asia Pac J Clin Nutr* 2004; 13(2): 217–20

29. Vidal-Valverde, C *et al.* 'Changes in the carbohydrate composition of legumes after soaking and cooking', *J Am Diet Assoc* 1993; 93(5): 547–50

30. El Tiney, A H 'Proximate Composition and Mineral and Phytate Contents of Legumes Grown in Sudan', *Journal of Food Composition and Analysis* 1989; 2: 67–8

31. Rackis, J J *et al.* 'The USDA trypsin inhibitor study. I. Background, objectives and procedural details,' *Qualification of Plant Foods in Human Nutrition* 1985; 35

32. Rackis, J J 'Biological and physiological Factors in Soybeans,' *Journal of the American Oil Chemists' Society* Jan 1974; 51: 161–70

33. Divi, R L *et al.* 'Anti-thyroid isoflavones from the soybean,' *Biochemical Pharmacology* 1997; 54: 1087–96

34. Gikas, P D *et al.* 'Phytoestrogens and the risk of breast cancer: a review of the literature', *Int J Fertil Women's Med* 2005; 50(6): 250–8

35. White, L. 'Association of High Midlife Tofu Consumption with Accelerated Brain Aging', Plenary Session 8: Cognitive Function. The Third International Soy Symposium, Program, November 1999: 26

36. www.cspinet.org/new/200208121.html

37. www.cspinet.org/quorn/

38. Hoppe, C *et al.* 'Protein intake at 9 mo of age is associated with body size but not with body fat in 10–y-old Danish children', *Am J Clin Nutr* 2004; 79(3): 494–501

39. Obeid, R *et al.* 'The impact of vegetarianism on some haematological parameters', *Eur J Haematol* 2002; 69(5–6): 275–9

40. Hunt, J R. 'Bioavailability of iron, zinc, and other trace minerals from vegetarian diets', *Am J Clin Nutr* 2003; 78(3 Suppl): 633S-639S

41. Krajcovicova-Kudlackova, M *et al.* 'Iodine deficiency in vegetarians and vegans', *Ann Nutr Metab* 2003; 47(5): 183–5

42. Key, T J *et al.* 'Mortality in British vegetarians: review and preliminary results from EPIC-Oxford, *Am J Clin Nutr* 2003; 78(suppl): 533S-8S

43. Key, T J A *et al.* 'Dietary habits and mortality in 11,000 vegetarians and health-conscious people: results of a 17-year follow up', *BMJ* 1996; 313: 775–9

44. Thorogood, M *et al.* 'Risk of death from cancer and ischemic heart disease in meat and non-meat eaters', *BMJ* 1994; 308: 1667–70

Chapter 10

1. Borghi, L *et al.* 'Urinary volume, water and recurrences idiopathic calcium nephrolithiasis: a 5-year randomised prospective study', *Urology* 1996; 155: 839–43

2. Hughes, J *et al.* 'Diet and calcium stones', *Can Med Assoc J* 1992; 146: 137–43

3. Iguchi, M *et al.* 'Clinical effects of prophylactic dietary treatment on renal stones', *J Urology* 1990; 144: 229–32

4. Embon, O M *et al.* 'Chronic dehydration stone disease', *Br J Urology* 1990; 66: 357–62

5. Wilkens, L R *et al.* 'Risk factors for lower urinary tract cancer: the role of total fluid consumption, nitrites and nitrosamines, and selected foods', *Cancer Epidemiol Biomarkers Prev* 1996; 5: 116–66

6. Shannon, J *et al.* 'Relationship of food groups and water intake to colon cancer risk', *Cancer Epidemiol Biomarkers Prev* 1996; 5: 495–502

7. Chan, J *et al.* 'Water, other fluids, and fatal coronary heart disease: the Adventist Health Study', *Am J Epidemiol* 2002; 155(9): 827–33

8. Armstrong, L E *et al.* 'Urinary indices of hydration status', *Int J Sport Nutr* 1994; 4: 265–79

9. Robert, D *et al.* 'Chlorination, Chlorination By-Products, and Cancer: A Meta-Analysis', *American Journal of Public Health* 1992; 82(7): 955–63

10. Cantor, K P *et al.* 'Drinking Water Source and Chlorination By-products in Iowa. III. Risk of Brain Cancer', *Am J Epidemiol* 1999; 150(6): 552–60

11. Suay, Llopis L *et al.* 'Review of studies on exposure to aluminum and Alzheimer's disease', *Rev Esp Salud Pública* 2002; 76(6): 645–58

12. McDonagh, M *et al.* 'Systematic Review of Water Fluoridation', *BMJ* 2000; 321: 855–9

13. Schoppen, S *et al.* 'A Sodium-Rich Carbonated Mineral Water Reduces Cardiovascular Risk in Postmenopausal Women', *J Nutr* 2004; 134: 1058–63

14. Elliott, S S *et al.* 'Fructose, weight gain, and the insulin resistance syndrome', *Am J Clin Nutr* 2002; 76: 911–22

15. Gardner, E J *et al.* 'Black tea – helpful or harmful? A review of the evidence', *Eur J Clin Nutr* 2006 July 19 [Epub ahead of print]

16. Steptoe, A *et al.* 'The effects of tea on psychophysiological stress responsivity and post-stress recovery: a randomised double-blind trial', *Psychopharmacology* 23 September 2006 [Epub]

17. Cabrera, C *et al.* 'Beneficial effects of green tea – a review', *J Am Coll Nutr* 2006; 25(2): 79–99

18. Ibid.

19. Greenberg, J A *et al.* 'Coffee, diabetes and weight control', *Am J Clin Nutr* 2006; 84: 682–93

20. Hino, A *et al.* 'Habitual coffee but not green tea consumption is inversely associated with metabolic syndrome: An epidemiological study in a general Japanese population', *Diabetes Res Clin Pract* 2006 Oct 27 [Epub ahead of print]

21. Andersen, L F *et al.* 'Consumption of coffee is associated with reduced risk of death attributed to inflammatory and cardiovascular diseases in the Iowa Women's Health Study', *Am J Clin Nutr* 2006; 83(5): 1039–46

22. Bidel, S *et al.* 'Coffee consumption and risk of total and cardiovascular mortality among patients with type 2 diabetes', *Diabetologia* 2006; 49(11): 2618–26

23. White, I R *et al.* 'Alcohol consumption and mortality: modelling risks for men and women at different ages', *BMJ* 2002; 325: 191

24. McCann, S E *et al.* 'Alcoholic beverage preference and characteristics of drinkers and nondrinkers in western New York (United States)', *Nutr Metab Cardiovasc Dis* 2003; 13(1): 2–11

25. Tjonneland, A M *et al.* 'The connection between food and alcohol intake habits among 48,763 Danish men and women. A cross-sectional study in the project "Food, cancer and health"', *Ugeskr Laeger* 1999; 161(50): 6923–7

26. Barefoot, J C *et al.* 'Alcohol beverage preference, diet and health habits in the UNC Alumni Heart Study', *Am J Clin Nutr* 2002; 76(2): 466–72

Chapter 11

1. Jenkins, D J *et al.* 'Nibbling versus gorging: advantages of increased meal frequency', *N Engl J Med* 1989; 321(14): 929–34

2. Rashidi, M R *et al.* 'Effects of nibbling and gorging on lipid profiles, blood glucose and insulin levels in healthy subjects', *Saudi Med J* 2003; 24(9): 945–8
3. Jenkins, D J *et al.* 'Nibbling versus gorging: advantages of increased meal frequency', *N Engl J Med* 1989; 321(14): 929–34
4. Farschi, R H *et al.* 'Beneficial metabolic effects of regular meal frequency on dietary thermogenesis, insulin sensitivity, and fasting lipid profiles in healthy obese women', *Am J Clin Nutr* 2005; 81(1): 16–24
5. Speechly, D P *et al.* 'Acute appetite reduction associated with an increased frequency of eating in obese males', *International Journal of Obesity and Related Metabolic Disorders* 1999; 23(11): 1151–9
6. de Castro, J M 'The time of day of food intake influences overall intake in humans', *Journal of Nutrition* 2004; 134: 104–11
7. Ruidavets, J B *et al.* 'Eating frequency and body fatness in middle-aged men', *Int J Obesity* 2002; 26(11): 1476–83
8. Fabry, P *et al.* 'The frequency of meals and its relationship to overweight, hyper-cholesteremia, and decreased glucose-tolerance', *Lancet* 1964; 2: 614–15
9. Ibid.
10. Fabry, P *et al.* 'Meal frequency and ischaemic heart disease', *Lancet* 1968; 2: 190–1

Chapter 12

1. Yancy, W S Jr *et al.* 'A low carbohydrate, ketogenic diet versus a low-fat diet to treat obesity and hyperlipidemia. A randomized, controlled trial', *Ann Intern Med* 2004; 140: 69–77
2. Seidell, J C *et al.* 'Fasting respiratory exchange ratio and resting metabolic rate as predictors of weight gain: The Baltimore Longitudinal Study on Aging', *Int J Obesity* 1992; 16: 667–74
3. Froidevaux, F *et al.* 'Energy expenditure in obese women before and during weight loss, after refeeding, and in the weight-relapse period', *Am J Clin Nutr* 1993; 57: 35–42
4. Larson, D E *et al.* 'Energy metabolism in weight-stable post-obese individuals', *Am J Clin Nutr* 1995; 62: 735–9
5. Ferraro, R T *et al.* 'Relationship between skeletal muscle lipoprotein lipase activity and 24–hour macronutrient oxidation', *J Clin Invest* 1993; 92: 441–5
6. Zurlo, F *et al.* 'Whole-body energy metabolism and skeletal muscle biochemical characteristics', *Metabolism* 1994; 43: 481–6

7. Cooling, J *et al.* 'Differences in energy expenditure and substrate oxidation between habitual high fat and low fat consumers (phenotypes)', *International Journal of Obesity and Related Metabolic Disorders* 1998; 22(7): 612–18

8. Marrades, M P *et al.* 'Differences in short-term metabolic responses to a lipid load in lean (resistant) vs obese (susceptible) young male subjects with habitual high-fat consumption', *Eur J Clin Nutr* 2006 Aug 9 [Epub ahead of print]

9. Marques-Lopes, I *et al.* 'Postprandial de novo lipogenesis and metabolic changes induced by a high-carbohydrate, low-fat meal in lean and overweight men', *Am J Clin Nutr* 2001; 73(2): 253–62

10. Cooling, J *et al.* 'Are high-fat and low-fat consumers distinct phenotypes? Differences in the subjective and behavioural response to energy and nutrient challenges', *Eur J Clin Nutr* 1998; 52(3): 193–201

11. Blundell, J E *et al.* 'Routes to obesity: phenotypes, food choices and activity', *British Journal of Nutrition* 2000; 83 (suppl 1): S33–38

Chapter 16

1. Weyer, C *et al.* 'Energy metabolism after 2 y of energy restriction: the biosphere 2 experiment', *Am J Clin Nutr* 2000; 72(4): 946–53

Appendix D

1. McMillan, M *et al.* 'Preliminary observations on the effect of dietary Brussels sprouts on thyroid function', *Hum Toxicol* 1986; 5(1): 15–19

Index

This index is in word by word order. Page numbers in italics indicate tables and diagrams. Individual recipes are not included

blood tests
  for adrenal function 245–6
  for food intolerance 225, 226–7
  for hypothyroidism 253–4
body
  biochemical stability 25, 121–2, 175
  energy production 128–9
  percentage of water 107
body shape 137, 140
body temperature 140, 141
bone marrow, early man 2
bones 52–3, 112
brain
  early man 2–3
  effect of gluten 37–8, 56
  importance of water 107
  and omega-3 fats 93
  effect of opioid peptides 55–6
bread, GI *27*
breakfast 164, 165, 166, 167, 168
breakfast cereals *27*
brown rice 39
butter 55, 63, 80, 81

caffeine 116–17, 120, 139, 141
calcium, and dairy products 51–2
calorie consumption 66–7
calorie principle 66, 68
cancer
  and chlorinated water 111
  colon 90–1
  and fruit and vegetables 95
  green tea reducing risk 115
  and legumes 98–9
  effect of trans fat 61–2
  and water intake 108–9
Candida (fungal infection) 233–5
carbohydrates 21, *26–31*, 32–4, 67–8
carbonated water 113
cardiovascular disease
  and coffee 116
  and eggs 91–2

and frequency of meals 125
and fruit and vegetables 96
and nuts 97
and saturated fats 71–9, 82
and tea 115
and trans fat 61
and vegetarianism 103–4
and water 109, 113
carnitine 88
casein 54, 56, 225
cereals *see* breakfast cereals; grain
cerebral oedema 110
chewing 229–30
chicken, production 88–9
chimpanzees, diet 1
chlorine, in water processing 111
cholesterol 24, 34, 74–9, 83
'cis' fats 61
climate, and food availability 6, 128
coenzyme Q10 78
coffee 116, 119, 155, 156, 164
colon cancer 90–1
colonialists, diet and health 12
constipation 108
contamination of fish 93
cortisol 122, 240, 242, 244, 247
crackers, GI *27*
cruciferous vegetables 95, 255
cytotoxic tests 226

dairy products 4, 16, 51–6
  for 'gatherers' 157, *163*
  for 'hunter-gatherers' 156, *161*
  for 'hunters' 154, *159*
decaffeination processes 117
dehydration 108, 119
dental decay, Neolithic age 9
dental fluorosis 112
DHA 93
DHEA 240, 244, 247
di-iodotyrosine 257
diabetes 24

Notes

Notes

Notes

For more information and support, and to sign up for Dr Briffa's free daily True You tips and motivators delivered straight to your email inbox go to **www.thetrueyoudiet.com.**

Dr John Briffa can be contacted at:

Woolaston House
25 Southwood Lane
Highgate
London
N6 5ED
UK

Tel.: +44 (0) 208 341 3422
Fax: +44 (0) 208 340 1376

For Dr John Briffa's health-focused blog,
and to sign up for his free weekly e-newsletter, see
www.drbriffa.com

Titles of related interest

Ask and It Is Given
by Esther and Jerry Hicks

Earth Wisdom
by Glennie Kindred

Energy Secrets
by Alla Svirinskaya

Heal Your Body
by Louise L. Hay

The Power of Intention
by Wayne W. Dyer

What Are You Really Eating?
by Amanda Ursell

You Can Heal Your Life
by Louise L. Hay

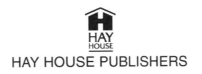

We hope you enjoyed this Hay House book.
If you would like to receive a free catalogue featuring additional
Hay House books and products, or if you would like information
about the Hay Foundation, please contact:

Hay House UK Ltd
292B Kensal Rd • London W10 5BE
Tel: (44) 20 8962 1230; Fax: (44) 20 8962 1239
www.hayhouse.co.uk

***

Published and distributed in the United States of America by:
Hay House, Inc. • PO Box 5100 • Carlsbad, CA 92018-5100
Tel: (1) 760 431 7695 or (800) 654 5126;
Fax: (1) 760 431 6948 or (800) 650 5115
www.hayhouse.com

Published and distributed in Australia by:
Hay House Australia Ltd • 18/36 Ralph St • Alexandria NSW 2015
Tel: (61) 2 9669 4299; Fax: (61) 2 9669 4144
www.hayhouse.com.au

Published and distributed in the Republic of South Africa by:
Hay House SA (Pty) Ltd • PO Box 990 • Witkoppen 2068
Tel/Fax: (27) 11 706 6612 • orders@psdprom.co.za

Distributed in Canada by:
Raincoast • 9050 Shaughnessy St • Vancouver, BC V6P 6E5
Tel: (1) 604 323 7100; Fax: (1) 604 323 2600

***

Sign up via the Hay House UK website to receive the Hay House
online newsletter and stay informed about what's going on with
your favourite authors. You'll receive bimonthly announcements
about discounts and offers, special events, product highlights,
free excerpts, giveaways, and more!
www.hayhouse.co.uk